Cardiovascular Hemorheology

SYOTEN OKA
Director of the National Cardiovascular Center Research Institute, Osaka, Japan

Cardiovascular Hemorheology

CAMBRIDGE UNIVERSITY PRESS
Cambridge
London   New York   New Rochelle
Melbourne   Sydney

Published by the Press Syndicate of the University of Cambridge
The Pitt Building, Trumpington Street, Cambridge CB2 1RP
32 East 57th Street, New York, NY 10022, USA
296 Beaconsfield Parade, Middle Park, Melbourne 3206, Australia.

© Cambridge University Press 1981

First published 1981

Printed in Great Britain at the University Press, Cambridge

British Library cataloguing in publication data

Oka, Syoten
Cardiovascular hemorheology
1. Blood – Circulation
I. Title
612'.13   QP102   80-41338
ISBN 0 521 23650 9

This book is dedicated to
The late Mr Uneo Kobayashi

CONTENTS

	Preface	xi
1	**Introduction**	**1**
1.1	Rheology	1
1.2	Biorheology	2
1.3	Cardiovascular hemorheology	3
2	**Rheological concepts**	**5**
2.1	Solid and fluid	5
2.2	Newtonian and non-Newtonian flow	7
2.3	Laminar flow in a cylindrical tube	10
2.4	Turbulent flow	13
2.5	Suspensions	15
2.6	Hookean solid	19
2.7	Viscoelasticity	20
2.8	Strain energy density function	24
2.9	Thixotropy	26
3	**Blood rheology**	**28**
3.1	Blood	28
3.2	Aggregation of red cells	29
3.3	Sedimentation of red cells	31
3.4	Non-Newtonian viscosity	33
3.5	Thixotropy and viscoelasticity	34
3.6	Factors affecting blood viscosity	38
3.7	Casson fluid	40
3.8	Plasma layer	46
3.9	Radial migration	48
3.10	Flow of red cell suspensions in small tubes	51
3.11	Fahraeus effect	54
3.12	Fahraeus–Lindqvist effect	55
3.13	Wall surface effect—Copley–Scott Blair phenomenon	57
3.14	Disturbed flows of red cell suspensions	60
3.15	Viscosity of blood clots	60
3.16	Blood rheology at near-zero gravity	63
3.17	Blood rheology and clinical medicine	65

Contents

4	**Red cell deformability**	**67**
4.1	Red cell deformability	67
4.2	Red cell morphology	68
4.3	Measuring techniques	73
4.4	Factors affecting red cell deformability	81
4.5	Significance of deformability in blood flow	84
4.6	Red cell deformability and clinical medicine	85
5	**Rheology of microcirculation**	**87**
5.1	Significance of rheology in microcirculation	87
5.2	Flow of plasma through capillaries	88
5.3	Flow of Casson fluid through a capillary	95
5.4	Capillary–tissue fluid exchange	98
5.5	Bolus flow	102
5.6	Sheet flow	106
5.7	Microcirculation and clinical medicine	108
6	**Rheology of blood vessels**	**111**
6.1	Blood vessel walls	111
6.2	Forces in blood vessel walls	114
6.3	General theory of circumferential tension	115
6.4	Stress distribution in blood vessel walls	120
6.5	Incremental theory of blood vessel walls	125
6.6	Nonlinear theory of elastic deformation	129
6.7	Tethering effect on the stresses in blood vessels	131
6.8	Some rheological models of blood vessels	134
7	**Pulsatile flow**	**138**
7.1	Pulse	138
7.2	Theoretical studies of pulse waves	139
7.3	Oscillatory flow in a rigid tube	141
7.4	Wave propagation in elastic tubes	143
7.5	Pressure–flow relationship	147
7.6	Pulsatile flow in microvessels	149
8	**Hemorheological aspects of cardiovascular diseases**	**151**
8.1	Flow in a locally constricted tube	151
8.2	Post-stenotic dilatation	157
8.3	Flow at branching sites	158
8.4	Thrombosis	160
8.5	Atherosclerosis	163
8.6	Protein uptake by arterial wall	167
8.7	Permeability and pathways of macromolecules	171
8.8	Physical theory of vascular permeability to proteins	175
8.9	Stresses in the arterial wall as a cause of permeability	184

8.10	Interaction of blood flow and arterial endothelium	187
9	**Prospects for cardiovascular hemorheology in the future**	**190**
	References	193
	Index	**206**

PREFACE

Since the establishment of the Society of Rheology in 1929, rheology as the science of deformation and flow of materials has been developed not only due to academic interest, but also to meet the needs of industry. Later, biorheology, the rheology of biological systems, began to develop rapidly. Particularly, to the biorheology of blood and blood vessels the name 'hemorheology' was given by Professor A. L. Copley.

This book attempts to describe systematically the basic concepts, facts and the present status of cardiovascular hemorheology. The significance of cardiovascular hemorheology is increasing, not only from the standpoint of physical sciences and engineering, but also from that of physiology, medicine and surgery. This book will serve partly as an introduction to cardiovascular hemorheology for beginners, but it will also be helpful to investigators doing further research.

Because cardiovascular hemorheology is a relatively new subject, and because of its multidisciplinary character, there are many problems which have not yet been clarified or generally accepted. I believe that the reader will become aware of the many problems which remain to be solved. This book is not simply a review of work done in cardiovascular hemorheology; I have attempted to give the reader a critical assessment with insight, which points the way ahead for further research.

It may be felt that I have quoted much of my own work. This is not because I am under any delusions that my work is better than that of other hemorheologists, but simply because I know it better than I know that of other people. I have also quoted some of my colleagues in Japan because their work seems less accessible to most investigators elsewhere in the world.

I have tried to emphasize theoretical aspects rather than purely experimental or practical aspects, and to introduce as many recent important works as possible, but to my regret many works could not be covered because of the limited space.

I feel greatly honored to have been asked by Dr Alan Winter of Cambridge University Press to write a book on Cardiovascular Hemorheology, an extremely charming title. My sincere thanks are also due to Mr Hideyuki Niimi, Ph.D. and Mr Takashi Yamakawa, M.D. at our Research Institute for their valuable advice and patient help in preparing the manuscript. Without their assistance it would never have been completed.

I am most grateful to the following for permission to copy figures and tables from their publications and to the authors whose names are cited in the legends: Academic Press, Figs. 25, 31, 33, 36, 49, 73, 74, 78 and 92; American Heart Association, Figs. 62 and 80; Birkhäuser Verlag, Fig. 46; Cambridge University Press, Fig. 51; Dr Dietrich Steinkopff Verlag, Fig. 27; Elsevier/North-Holland Biomedical Press, Figs. 26 and 28; Excerpta Medica, Figs. 81, 82 and 83; F.K. Schattauer Verlag GmbH, Fig. 43; HP Publishing Co., Fig. 34; Japanese College of Angiology, Fig. 77; Macmillan Journals Ltd, Fig. 19; Mrs Renee McDonald, Fig. 69; Oxford University Press, Fig. 86; Pergamon Press, Figs. 5, 14, 15, 17, 18, 21, 22, 23, 29, 30, 40, 48, 50, 52, 55, 58, 59, 60, 61, 63, 70, 71, 72, 75, 76, 79, 84, 88 and 90; Springer-Verlag, Figs. 32, 35, 38, 39 and 41; The American Physiological Society, Figs. 24, 54, 85 and Table 3; The Institute of Physics, Fig. 68; The Japan Society of Applied Physics, Fig. 44; The Journal of Physiology, Fig. 67; The Physiological Society of Japan, Figs. 64 and 65; The Rockefeller University Press, Fig. 87; The Society of Rheology, Fig. 16; Year Book Medical Publishers, Fig. 1.

The author wishes to acknowledge his indebtedness to Cambridge University Press and especially to Mr Robin Rees and Miss Jayne Matthews for their unfailing cooperation.

National Cardiovascular Center
Research Institute
Osaka, Japan

Syoten Oka
March, 1980

1

Introduction

1.1 Rheology

About 1920, an American physico-chemist called Bingham became interested in the flow properties of such materials as paint, clay paste, and printing ink, and drew attention to the importance of the science of the deformation and flow of materials. As a result, the American Society of Rheology was established in 1929. 'Rheo' is Greek for 'flow', so Bingham called the science of the deformation and flow of materials '*rheology*'. The word 'flow' may be defined as a deformation proceeding irreversibly with time.

Since we already have the classical theory of elasticity for the deformation of elastic bodies, and classical fluid mechanics for the flow of fluids, rheology may seem unnecessary. But this is not so. The classical theory of elasticity is based on *Hooke's law*, i.e. strain is proportional to stress; and classical fluid mechanics is based on *Newton's law of viscosity*, i.e. shear rate is proportional to shear stress. However, many everyday materials do not obey these laws.

Generally, the relationship between the strain and the stress for a given material is called the *constitutive equation* of the material. Here the words strain and stress should be interpreted in the broadest sense to include their time derivatives.

The theories of elasticity and fluid mechanics lay emphasis on equilibrium and motion, while rheology is more comprehensive. Since this comprehensive view reflects the variety and individuality of materials, the relationship between mechanical properties and their structures is of great importance in rheology. Since rheology is concerned with individual materials, it is primarily an experimental discipline, but theories have also been developed to cover both phenomenological and molecular aspects.

Rheology is of great practical importance. All industries dealing with ceramics, rubber, plastics, fiber, paint, and food have processes which involve the deformation and flow of such materials. Rheology was developed originally to meet the requirements of industry.

Thus rheology, like cybernetics, is very broad in scope, and is involved in many fields of science. It is closely linked to physics (particularly materials science, and mechanics) and chemistry (particularly colloid chemistry, polymer chemistry, and industrial chemistry).

1.2   Biorheology

With the development of rheology, much attention has recently been paid to the rheology of biological systems. This field is called *biorheology*, and is in the borderland between rheology and biology or medicine. Biorheology deals with rheological phenomena in living organisms, and the rheological properties of substances constituting living organisms. Examples of subjects dealt with in biorheology are: flow properties of biofluids (blood, lymph, synovial fluid, cerebrospinal and intra-ocular fluid, sputum, saliva, cervical mucus), protoplasmic streaming, deformation of cells (red blood cells, sea urchin eggs), deformation of soft tissues (blood vessels, muscles, heart, bladder, mesentery, eye lens, cartilage), bone, and also solutions of proteins, nucleic acids and polysaccharides. Much attention has recently been paid to the relation between rheological properties of biological systems and their biological functions. Just as rheology has been developed to meet the requirements of industry, biorheology has been developed to meet those of medicine and biology.

By far the largest amount of biorheological work has been done on blood and blood vessels. This area of biorheology is called *hemorheology*. Originally, in 1952, it was defined by Copley as 'rheological properties of cellular and plasmatic components of blood in macroscopic, microscopic, and submicroscopic dimensions, and the rheological properties of vessel structure with which blood comes into direct contact'. How hemodynamics differs from hemorheology can best be explained by comparing fluid mechanics and rheology.

Hemorheology is important in both basic and clinical medicine. It may contribute to rapid progress in medical understanding of blood circulation.

1.3 Cardiovascular Hemorheology

The circulatory system transports and distributes essential substances to the tissues and removes the by-products of metabolism. It also plays an important role in regulating body temperature, transporting humors around the body, and adjusting supplies of oxygen and nutrients.

The *cardiovascular system* consists of a pump, a series of distributing and collecting tubes, and a system of microvessels that permit rapid exchange between the tissues and the vascular channels. Figure 1 shows a grossly simplified diagram of the parallel and series arrangement of the vessels comprising the cardiovascular system.

The heart is made up of two pumps in series: one to propel blood through the lungs to exchange oxygen and carbon dioxide (the pulmonary circulation). The other to propel blood to all other tissues of the body (the systemic circulation). The flow through the heart is made unidirectional by flap valves.

While the cardiac output is intermittent, the flow to the periphery is continuous. This is due to the distension of both the aorta and its branches during ventricular contraction (systole). The elastic deformation of the wall of large arteries recovers during ventricular relaxation (diastole), which results in forward propulsion of blood.

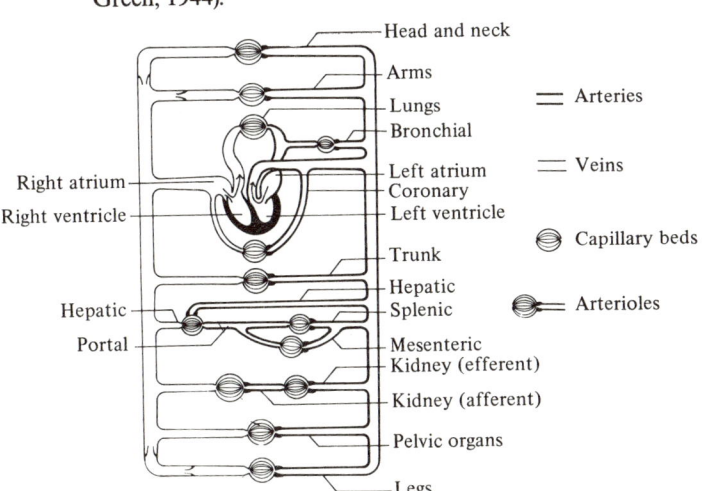

Fig. 1. Schematic diagram of the circulatory system (From Green, 1944).

From a predominantly elastic structure, the aorta, the peripheral arteries become more muscular until at the arterioles the muscular layer predominates. The arterioles are the principal points of resistance to blood flow in the circulatory system. The contraction of the muscle of the arterioles regulates blood flow through the tissues and blood pressure in the arteries. While blood pressure is reduced by the arterioles, the pulsatile character of arterial blood flow is eliminated at the capillary level and changes to a steady flow. Since the walls of capillaries are only one cell thick and since blood flows very slowly there, it is very easy for blood and tissue to exchange substances.

Blood entering the right ventricle via the right atrium is pumped through the pulmonary arterial system, carbon dioxide being released and oxygen taken in through the lung capillaries. The oxygen-rich blood returns via the pulmonary veins to the left atrium and ventricle to complete the cycle.

In blood circulation, blood rheology is most important in *microvessels* i.e. arterioles, capillaries, and venules, where the specific rheological properties come into play most markedly. The capacity of a red blood cell to deform under a mechanical force is referred to as its *deformability*. Red blood cell deformability plays a significant role in blood circulation. It allows the passage of red cells through capillaries with diameters smaller than that of a red cell at rest. Any vessel that allows an exchange of substances through its wall is called an exchange vessel. This process mainly occurs in microvessels. The exchange of substances occurs by one of the three major mechanisms, i.e. diffusion, bulk flow, or vesicular transport. Detailed descriptions of microcirculation, red cell deformability and vascular permeability are given later.

2

Rheological concepts

This chapter provides a brief résumé of basic concepts which are most important in hemorheology. As with all rapidly growing subjects, definitions can only be as precise as current knowledge allows. Space is limited, and we cannot discuss concepts as fully as we would like. For concepts or technical terms which are not of central importance, we have tried to give brief definitions or illustrations as they arise.

2.1 Solid and fluid

(*a*) *Stress and strain*

Let us consider a solid which is in equilibrium under external forces (Fig. 2). Imagine an arbitrary plane element at any point inside the body. Then forces will be exerted on both sides of the plane. In general, these forces will be at some angle to the plane. These forces will of course be equal and opposite. Each force can be resolved into a normal (or perpendicular) component, and into a tangential (or shear) component. If the area of the plane element is very small, then the ratios of these forces to the area are independent of the area of the plane element. These ratios are respectively called the *normal stress* and *tangential stress*.

If the orientation of the plane element be changed, without changing the position, then the values of the normal stress and tangential stress will be changed. It can be demonstrated that there are three orientations of the plane element for which the tangential stresses vanish, and that the three orientations are perpendicular to each other. Furthermore, it can be shown that the sum of the three normal stresses does not change its value with change in orientation of the plane element. That is, the sum of the three normal stresses is a *stress invariant*. The arithmetical mean of the three normal stresses is called the *hydrostatic pressure* or hydrostatic tension when the mean is negative or positive. The units of the normal stress, the tangential stress or the hydrostatic pressure are dyn cm^{-2} in the CGS (centimeter–gram–second) system.

When the shape or size of a body is changed, the body is said to undergo a *deformation*. Let us consider a small rectangular element in an undeformed body. In the deformed body, the lengths of the sides and the angles generally change, and the element is said to undergo a strain. In particular, if all points in the body are in the same state of strain, a body is said to undergo a homogeneous deformation.

(b) *Mechanical criterion for solid and fluid*

Tangential stress does not generally vanish in a deformed solid, whereas it always vanishes in a fluid at rest. This is the criterion of continuum mechanics for distinguishing between a solid and a

Fig. 2. Stress (*a*) and deformation (*b*).

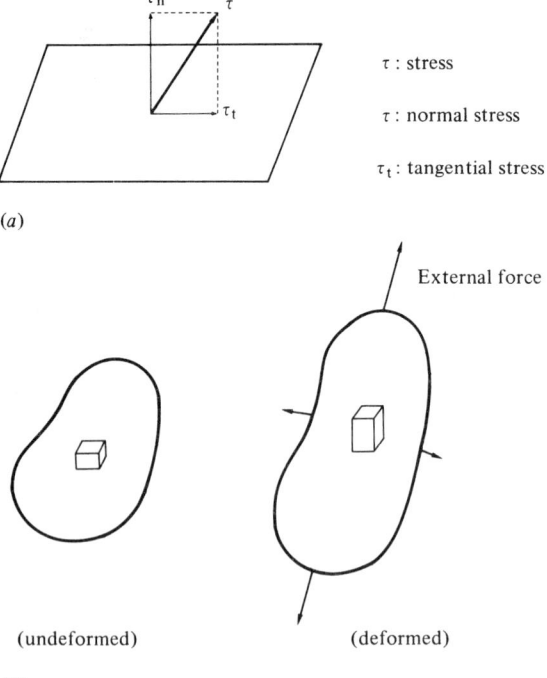

fluid. Thus, a fluid shows no resistance to change of shape, whereas a solid generally keeps its own shape under its weight.

Tangential stress appears when a fluid flows. This means that the fluid has *viscosity*. In continuum mechanics a fluid has *compressibility* besides viscosity. The compressibility is related to the normal stress in a fluid at rest, while the viscosity is related to the tangential stress in a fluid in motion.

It is important to distinguish between solid and fluid when considering certain bodies such as soft plastics. If such a body is deformed rapidly, it behaves as a solid; and if it is deformed slowly, it behaves as a fluid. At sufficiently low temperatures it behaves as in a glassy state, while at higher temperatures it sometimes behaves as a fluid.

(c) *Structural criterion for solid and fluid*

The distinction between solid and fluid states can be made from a different, structural point of view. For example, water shows a phase transition at 0 °C under one atmosphere pressure. Solid ice exists below 0 °C, while liquid water exists above 0 °C. In general, crystalline substances are solids. Some solid polymeric substances, however, gradually soften on heating until they become a fluid without having a precise melting point.

2.2 Newtonian and non-Newtonian flow

(a) *Newtonian flow*

Suppose that a fluid is confined between two parallel plates A and B whose distance h is very small (Fig. 3). If the plate

Fig. 3. Couette flow.

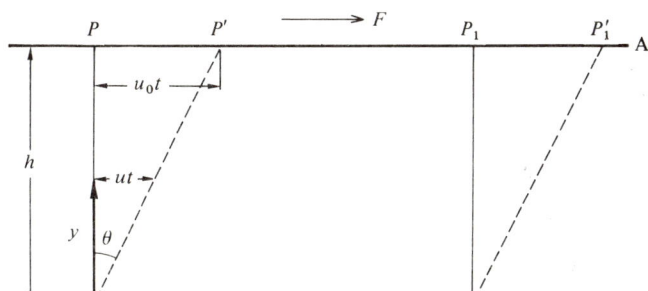

B is fixed and a constant tangential force F is applied to the plate A, the tangential force per unit area acting upon it is equal to F/S, where S is the surface area of the fluid in contact with the plate. Then, the flow velocity of the fluid, u, at any point is proportional to its vertical distance y from the plate B:

$$u = Dy \qquad (2.1)$$

where D is a constant. It can generally be accepted that the fluid does not slip at the plates. Then, if we denote the velocity of the plate A by u_0, we have

$$u_0 = Dh \quad \text{or} \quad D = u_0/h \qquad (2.2)$$

Since D represents the ratio of the relative velocity to their distance, it is called the *velocity gradient*. The flow of fluid between two parallel plates is generally called the *Couette flow*.

In the Couette flow, the fluid initially contained in the rectangular region OPP_1O_1 is deformed into the parallelepiped $OP'P'_1O_1$ at time t. Such a deformation is called *shear*, and is represented by:

$$\gamma = \tan \theta \qquad (2.3)$$

with $\theta = \angle POP'$. Since $PP' = u_0 t$, we have

$$\gamma = \tan \theta = u_0 t/h = Dt \qquad (2.4)$$

or

$$\dot{\gamma} = D \qquad (2.5)$$

Here the dot over the letter represents the derivative with respect to time: $\dot{\gamma} = d\gamma/dt$. The quantity $\dot{\gamma}$ is called the *shear rate* (or the rate of shear), and is equal to the velocity gradient in the Couette flow. Since γ is a dimensionless quantity, the shear rate is measured in s^{-1} in CGS units.

Let us consider an arbitrary plane which is parallel to the plate in the Couette flow. The upper part of the fluid exerts a tangential force in the opposite direction. The tangential force per unit area, τ, within the fluid is called the *shear stress*, and is given by:

$$\tau = F/S \qquad (2.6)$$

There is a close relationship between the shear rate and the shear stress. The simplest relationship is Newton's law of viscosity; the

2.2 Newtonian and non-Newtonian flow

velocity gradient is proportional to the shear stress:

$$D = \tau/\eta \tag{2.7}$$

where η is the *Newtonian viscosity*. A fluid which obeys Newton's law of viscosity is called a *Newtonian fluid*, and its flow is called a *Newtonian flow*. In a Newtonian fluid, the viscosity is a material constant which depends only upon the temperature. From Eqs. (2.5) and (2.7), we have the relation:

$$\eta = \tau/\dot{\gamma} \tag{2.8}$$

(b) Non-Newtonian flow

A fluid which does not obey Newton's law of viscosity is called a *non-Newtonian fluid*. The rheological behavior of a fluid is specified by the flow curve:

$$\dot{\gamma} = f(\tau) \tag{2.9}$$

where $\dot{\gamma}$ is the *shear rate* and τ is the shear stress. In such a non-Newtonian fluid, the *apparent viscosity*, η_a, is defined as the ratio of the shear stress to the shear rate:

$$\eta_a = \tau/\dot{\gamma} \tag{2.10}$$

The apparent viscosity has the same units as the Newtonian viscosity, but it is not a material constant, because it depends upon the shear rate.

The relationship between the apparent viscosity and the shear rate can be divided into three groups (Fig. 4): (A) *shear-thinning*, i.e. a reduction of viscosity with increasing shear rate; (B) *shear-thickening*, i.e. an increase in viscosity with increasing shear rate; (C) Newtonian viscosity, which does not depend on the shear rate.

Fig. 4. Non-Newtonian behavior.

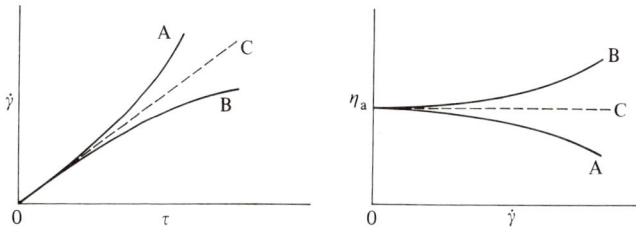

2.3 Laminar flow in a cylindrical tube

(a) *Laminar flow*

Let us consider a steady flow of fluid through a long cylindrical tube. When the flow velocity is not large, the fluid particles move parallel to the axis of the tube.

Now imagine that the fluid is composed of a number of thin cylindrical shells (Fig. 5). If the fluid does not slip at the wall, the shell in direct contact with the wall is at rest, but the shells move faster the nearer they are to the axis of the tube; the layers slide over each other without mixing. Such a flow is called *laminar flow*, or sometimes *telescopic flow*.

Let us denote by $u(r)$ the velocity of the fluid at a distance r from the axis of the tube; its functional form represents the *velocity distribution* or the *velocity profile* over a cross-section of the tube. The volume of fluid flowing across a cross-section per unit time is called the *flow rate*. The volume of fluid flowing across the annular region of width dr is $u \cdot 2\pi r dr$. Thus the flow rate Q is given by:

$$Q = \int_0^R u \cdot 2\pi r dr \tag{2.11}$$

where R is the radius of the tube. The mean velocity U over a cross-section is defined by

$$U = Q/\pi R^2 \tag{2.12}$$

(b) *Stokes' relation*

In order to maintain a steady flow through a cylindrical tube, a pressure difference along the length of the tube is necessary. Since there exists no radial motion, the pressure is constant over any cross-section.

Let us consider the cylinder of a fluid contained within a distance r of the axis of the tube, and having length L (Fig. 6). If we denote the longitudinal shear stress acting on the cylindrical surface by τ,

Fig. 5. Laminar flow in a cylindrical tube. (From Whitmore, 1968.)

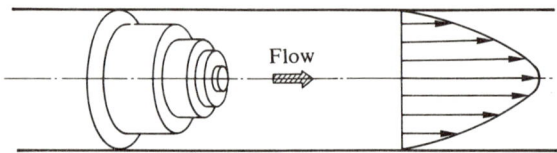

2.3 Laminar flow in a cylindrical tube

then the resultant force arising from the longitudinal tractions on the cylindrical surface becomes $2\pi r L\tau$. For Newtonian as well as non-Newtonian fluids, the net driving force is given by $\pi r^2 \Delta p$, where Δp is the pressure difference along the length L. Since the flow is steady, we have from the balance of forces $2\pi r L\tau = \pi r^2 \Delta p$, i.e.

$$\tau = \frac{\Delta p}{2L} r \qquad (2.13)$$

This is called *Stokes' relation*.

For a given pressure gradient, the shear stress is proportional to the distance from the axis. The shear stress vanishes at the axis, and is highest at the wall surface:

$$\tau_w = \frac{\Delta p}{2L} R \qquad (2.14)$$

Hence we have

$$\tau = \frac{r}{R} \tau_w \qquad (2.15)$$

(c) *Velocity distribution and flow rate*

For the steady laminar flow of a non-Newtonian fluid specified by the flow curve $f(\tau)$ through a rigid cylindrical tube, general formulas have been derived for velocity distribution, flow rate, and the shear rate.

(i) Velocity distribution

The shear rate is expressed in terms of $u(r)$ by $\dot{\gamma} = -du/dr$. Hence we have

$$-du/dr = f(\tau) \qquad (2.16)$$

Fig. 6. Diagram for Stokes' relation.

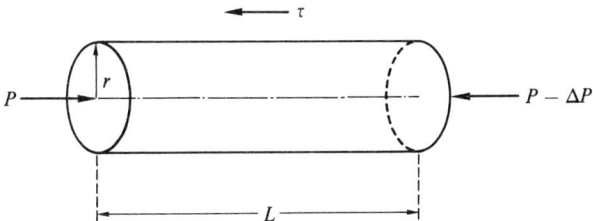

Changing the variable of integration from r to τ using Stokes' relation, Eq. (2.13), we obtain

$$u = \frac{R}{\tau_w} \int_{\tau}^{\tau_w} f(\tau) d\tau \qquad (2.17)$$

The above expression for u has been obtained as function of τ. If we use Stokes' relation, the velocity u can be expressed as a function of r.

(ii) Flow rate

By partial integration of Eq. (2.11) we obtain

$$Q = \frac{\pi R^3}{\tau_w^3} \int_0^{\tau_w} f(\tau) \tau^2 d\tau \qquad (2.18)$$

Since τ_w is given by Eq. (2.14), the flow rate Q is expressed as a function of the pressure gradient $\Delta p/L$. It should be noted that the no-slip condition at the wall has been used in the derivation of Eqs. (2.17) and (2.18).

(d) *Poiseuille flow*

The laminar flow of a Newtonian fluid in a straight circular tube is called the *Poiseuille flow*. Its velocity profile and flow rate can be obtained from the general formulas above.

(i) Velocity profile

The flow curve for a Newtonian fluid is:

$$f(\tau) = \tau/\eta \qquad (2.19)$$

Thus, substituting Eq. (2.19) into Eq. (2.17), we obtain

$$u = \frac{1}{4\eta} \frac{\Delta p}{L} (R^2 - r^2) \qquad (2.20)$$

As is well-known, the velocity profile becomes parabolic.

(ii) Flow rate

Substituting Eq. (2.19) into Eq. (2.18), we obtain *Poiseuille's law*

$$Q = \frac{\pi R^4}{8\eta} \frac{\Delta p}{L} \qquad (2.21)$$

The flow rate is not only proportional to the pressure gradient, but also proportional to the fourth power of the radius.

The graph Q–Δp is a straight line passing through the origin, and the viscosity η can be obtained from the inclination of the straight line.

(iii) Shear rate

The shear rate at the wall is given by $\dot{\gamma}_w = \tau_w/\eta$. Thus we have

$$\dot{\gamma}_w = \frac{1}{2\eta}\frac{\Delta p}{L}R \tag{2.22}$$

or

$$\dot{\gamma}_w = \frac{4Q}{\pi R^3} = \frac{4U}{R} \tag{2.23}$$

U being the mean velocity.

2.4 Turbulent flow

(a) *Critical Reynolds number*

The foregoing types of flow assumed laminar flow, i.e. adjacent layers of fluids would remain separate. Flow which is not laminar is called *turbulent flow*. In such a turbulent flow, no distinct layers are observed; all layers mix with one another by forming eddies and vortices. The most striking features of turbulent flow are that the velocity and pressure at a fixed point in space fluctuate very irregularly, and rapidly.

Turbulent flow occurs when the flow rate exceeds a certain critical value, usually expressed as the *critical Reynolds number*. The *Reynolds number*, Re, is a dimensionless quantity; for Newtonian flow in a cylindrical tube of diameter D,

$$Re = \rho UD/\eta \tag{2.24}$$

where U is the fluid velocity averaged over the cross-sectional area, ρ is the density, and η is the viscosity of the fluid. The actual value of the critical Reynolds number, Re_c, is approximately 2300, but the value depends on the details of the experimental arrangement, in particular on the amount of disturbance suffered by the fluid before entering the tube.

It should be noted that the Reynolds number can be interpreted generally as the ratio of inertial force to frictional force. As is shown later, the Reynolds number plays an important role in distinguishing the flow in large arteries from that in microvessels. As mentioned earlier, the velocity profile for the steady laminar flow is parabolic, but the profile for turbulent flow becomes blunter, with a larger velocity gradient near the wall.

In a steady laminar flow of Newtonian fluids through a tube, the flow rate Q increases linearly with increase in the pressure gradient $\Delta p/L$. After the onset of turbulent flow, the flow rate increases with approximately the square root of the applied pressure gradient (Fig. 7). This indicates that the additional shear stress increases the number and size of eddies more than it increases the flow of the bulk of the fluid.

(b) *Coefficient of resistance*

We shall now consider fully developed turbulent flow in a cylindrical tube. Stokes' relation holds for turbulent flow as well as for laminar flow, and the shear stress τ reaches a maximum τ_w at the wall.

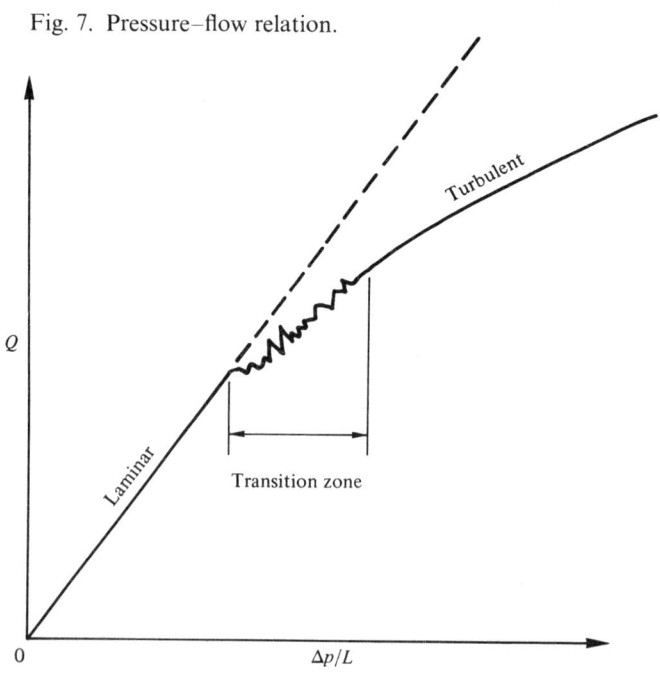

Fig. 7. Pressure–flow relation.

For laminar flow, Poiseuille's law provides a theoretical relationship between the flow rate and the pressure difference. For turbulent flow, however, no such theoretical relationship has yet been derived.

Let us define the *coefficient of resistance* λ by

$$\frac{\Delta p}{L} = \frac{\lambda}{D}\frac{1}{2}\rho U^2 \tag{2.25}$$

Since both the pressure drop Δp and $\frac{1}{2}\rho U^2$ ($U=$ flow velocity averaged over the cross-sectional area, $\rho=$ density) are measured as energy per unit volume, λ is dimensionless. Substituting the above equation into Eq. (2.14), we have

$$\tau_w = \tfrac{1}{8}\lambda\rho U^2 \tag{2.26}$$

The coefficient of resistance for a Poiseuille flow can easily be obtained. From Eqs. (2.21) and (2.25) we have

$$\pi R^2 U = \frac{\pi R^4}{8\eta}\frac{\lambda\rho U^2}{4R}$$

or

$$\lambda = \frac{64}{\rho U D/\eta} = \frac{64}{Re} \tag{2.27}$$

Blasius (1913) made a critical survey of numerous experimental results for turbulent flow, and he was able to establish the following empirical equation:

$$\lambda = 0.3164\left(\frac{\rho U D}{\eta}\right)^{-1/4} = \frac{0.3164}{Re^{0.25}} \tag{2.28}$$

This is valid for the frictional resistance of smooth tubes of circular cross-section, and is known as *Blasius' formula*. According to this result, λ is a function of the Reynolds number only. Blasius' formula is valid in the range of $Re < 100\,000$. The pressure drop in turbulent flow in that range is proportional to $U^{7/4}$, i.e. the mean velocity increases with the $\frac{4}{7}$th power of the pressure gradient.

2.5 Suspensions

(a) Viscosity

The fluid in which small particles are suspended is called a *suspension*. The viscosity of a suspension depends on various factors, such as the viscosity of the suspending medium, the concentration, the particle shape, the interaction between the particles, on whether the particles are rigid or deformable, and on the temperature.

The viscosity of a suspension always increases with the concentration. It is very important to show theoretically that the viscosity of a suspension is always greater than that of the corresponding medium. In order to explain this fact, it is helpful to realize that the viscosity of any fluid is associated with dissipation of mechanical energy into heat within the fluid.

Let us consider a Couette flow with the velocity gradient $D = u_0/h$, as in Sect. 2. The work done by the tangential force F on the fluid initially contained in the rectangular region OPP_1O_1 during the time dt is given by $Fu_0\,dt$. Then,

$$Fu_0\,dt = S\tau u_0\,dt = S\eta D u_0\,dt = Sh\eta D^2\,dt$$

using eqs. (2.2), (2.6) and (2.7). Thus, we know that the *dissipation of mechanical energy* w per unit volume per unit time is

$$w = \eta D^2 \tag{2.29}$$

Let us denote the viscosity of the suspending medium by η_0 and the dissipation of mechanical energy by w_0, the viscosity of the suspension by η_s and the dissipation of mechanical energy by w_0, the velocity gradient D being the same for the two cases. Then

Fig. 8. Couette flow around a rigid sphere.

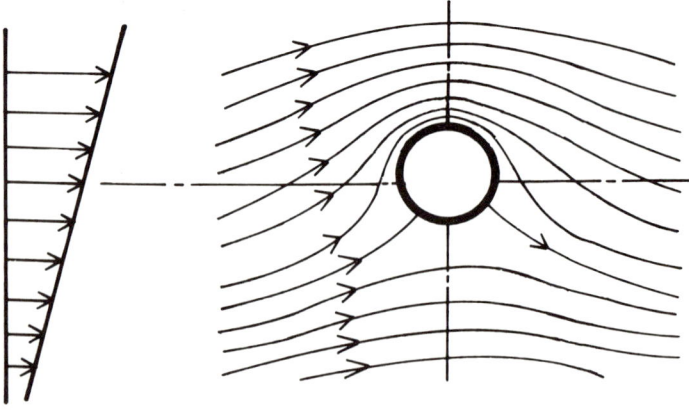

2.5 Suspensions

we have

$$w_0 = \eta_0 D^2 \qquad w_s = \eta_s D^2$$

When the particles are absent, the streamlines are parallel in the suspending medium, whereas in a suspension they take roundabout ways around the suspended particles (Fig. 8). This means that w_s is greater than w_0, or

$$\eta_s > \eta_0 \tag{2.30}$$

The concentration of a suspension is usually expressed by the *volume fraction* ϕ, which is defined as the ratio of the total volume of suspended particles to the total volume of the suspension. Here the volume of suspended particles includes the volume of the particles and also the volume of adsorbed fluid.

Einstein (1906) first found theoretically that the viscosity of the suspension η was related to that of the suspending medium η_0 at the same temperature by the equation

$$\eta = \eta_0(1 + 2.5\phi) \tag{2.31}$$

where ϕ is the volume fraction of the suspended particles. Equation (2.31) is called *Einstein's equation*. It was derived on the basis of the dissipation of energy mentioned above. It was derived under the following assumptions: (i) the suspended particles are large compared with the molecules of the suspending medium but small compared with the dimensions of the measuring apparatus; (ii) the suspended particles are spherical and rigid; (iii) the suspension is so dilute that no particle causes disturbance to the hydrodynamic flow of suspending medium past another particle; (iv) the effects of gravitation, and inertia and turbulence of the suspending medium are negligible.

Eirich, Bunzl & Margaretta (1936) tested Eq. (2.31) experimentally using small glass spheres, and demonstrated that the coefficient 2.5 was valid.

If the concentration of rigid spheres is increased above about $\phi = 0.01$, mutual interaction occurs between them, and the viscosity rises faster with the concentration than is predicted by Einstein's equation.

If the suspended particles are not spheres, but particles of other shapes such as ellipsoids or rods, the interaction forces are larger. The viscosity of such a suspension with small volume fraction is given by

$$\eta = \eta_0(1 + v\phi) \qquad (2.32)$$

where v is called the *form factor*, which is greater than 2.5 and increases with increasing asymmetry of the particles.

When the volume fraction becomes large, the particles interfere with one another, and Eqs. (2.31) and (2.32) are no longer valid. It becomes necessary to introduce terms of higher orders of ϕ.

Whether a suspension acts as a Newtonian or non-Newtonian fluid depends on the concentration and nature of the suspended particles. A suspension of rigid, non-interacting spheres at concentrations so low that mechanical interference can be ignored is Newtonian. However, there is some experimental evidence that non-Newtonian behavior develops in suspensions of spheres if a concentration of about 40% is exceeded.

For suspensions of liquid drops which remain spherical in shape due to surface tension, Taylor (1932) obtained a formula:

$$\eta = \eta_0(1 + 2.5\phi T) \qquad (2.33)$$

with

$$T = \frac{p + 0.4}{p + 1} \qquad p = \frac{\eta_i}{\eta_0} \qquad (2.34)$$

T is called the *Taylor factor* ($T < 1$). Here η_i is the viscosity of the drop, and ϕ is the volume fraction of drops. When the drops become effectively rigid ($\eta_i/\eta_0 \to \infty$), Eq. (2.33) reduces to Eq. (2.31). The viscosity of suspension of liquid drops is smaller than that of the suspension of rigid spheres for given values of η_0 and ϕ, as would be expected. The Taylor factor can be regarded as a reduction factor such that ϕT is the effective volume fraction for rigid spheres.

(b) Particle motion

The motion of particles suspended in viscous fluids has been observed in the stationary layer of suspensions. Goldsmith & Mason (1975) developed ingenious devices: counter-rotating cylinders, parallel discs for the Couette flow apparatus, a four-roller device for the hyperbolic shear flow apparatus. In flow through

2.6 Hookean solid

rigid, circular glass tubes the particles are followed along the vessel with the aid of a travelling microscope. With these devices it is possible to photograph and study the motion of individual suspended particles and the suspending fluid over sufficiently long periods. Goldsmith & Mason observed the motion of the suspended particles by matching refractive indices of the dispersed and suspending phases and inserting visible tracer particles into the otherwise transparent system. They studied suspensions of rigid spheres, discs and rods, deformable droplets, flexible fibers and filaments. Their studies are closely related to hemorheology. Since suspended particles in their experiments differ essentially from red blood cells, one must be very careful in applying the results to blood rheology.

2.6 Hookean solid

Let us suppose that a solid is deformed by external forces, i.e. it undergoes a change in size and shape. The material is elastic if the body returns to its original size and shape with the removal of the applied forces. The forces applied to the body do work, which is stored in the body as *strain energy*.

The strain is proportional to the stress in any elastic body unless the strain exceeds a certain limit. This is *Hooke's law*, and the stress: strain ratio is generally called the *elastic modulus*. There are three fundamental types of deformation: elongation, volume

Table 1. *Relationship between G, K, E and σ.*

	G, E	G, K	E, K	G, σ	E, σ	K, σ
E	–	$\dfrac{9GK}{3K+G}$	–	$2G(1+\sigma)$	–	$3K(1-2\sigma)$
G	–	–	$\dfrac{3EK}{9K-E}$	–	$\dfrac{E}{2(1+\sigma)}$	$\dfrac{3K(1-2\sigma)}{2(1+\sigma)}$
K	$\dfrac{EG}{3(3G-E)}$	–	–	$G\dfrac{2(1+\sigma)}{3(1-2\sigma)}$	$\dfrac{E}{3(1-2\sigma)}$	–
σ	$\dfrac{E}{2G}-1$	$\dfrac{3K-2G}{2(3K+G)}$	$\dfrac{1}{2}\left(1-\dfrac{E}{3K}\right)$	–	–	–

change, and shear. For elongation, the elastic modulus is known as *Young's modulus, E*. For volume change, the elastic modulus is known as the *bulk modulus, K*. For shear, the elastic modulus is known as the *shear modulus, G*.

Any isotropic elastic body can be specified in terms of two independent elastic moduli. If we denote *Poisson's ratio* by σ, then any two of the four quantities E, K, G, and σ can be expressed in terms of the other two quantities (Table 1).

2.7 Viscoelasticity

(a) Time effects

The concept of the Hookean elasticity is an idealization; the behavior of real materials is much more complicated. Some materials, especially when stretched fairly rapidly, show *hysteresis*, i.e. the return of a stress–strain curve to its origin by a different path (Fig. 9). The curve obtained as the length is decreased falls below that obtained as the length is increased (the *hysteresis loop* is clockwise). The area of the loop is equal to the energy lost in the specimen during the cycle. Hysteresis occurs because a certain time is necessary for the strain to reach its equilibrium value.

A similar time effect also arises in the measurement of the elastic modulus. The more rapidly the strains are produced, the greater the tension produced by a given strain.

(b) Viscoelasticity

It is possible to picture the time effects by considering the behavior of mechanical models. These usually consist of a spring and a dash pot. A spring obeys Hooke's law, so that the strain γ is proportional to the stress τ: $\gamma = \tau/G$. A dash pot obeys Newton's

Fig. 9. Hysteresis and Hooke's law.

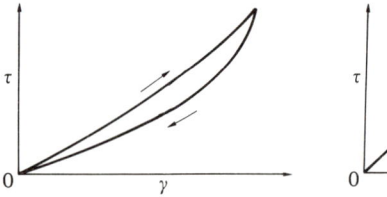

2.7 Viscoelasticity

law of viscosity, so that the strain rate $\dot{\gamma}$ is proportional to the stress: $\dot{\gamma} = \tau/\eta$.

A model in which a spring and a dash pot are connected in parallel is called a *Kelvin model* or a *Voigt model* (Fig. 10(a)). Since the two elements have the same strain, γ, and the stress in the Kelvin model is the sum of the stresses in the two elements, we have

$$\tau = G\gamma + \eta\dot{\gamma} \tag{2.35}$$

If a constant stress τ_0 is applied, we obtain

$$\gamma = \tau_0(1 - e^{-t/\tau'}) \tag{2.36}$$

where $\tau' = \eta/G$ is called the *retardation time*. The strain is delayed by the viscosity of the dash pot.

A model in which a spring and a dash pot are connected in series is called a *Maxwell model* (Fig. 10(b)). Since the two elements have the same stress, τ, and the strain in the Maxwell model is the sum of the strains in the two elements, we have

$$\dot{\gamma} = \frac{\dot{\tau}}{G} + \frac{\tau}{\eta} \tag{2.37}$$

If a constant strain, γ_0, is applied, we have

$$\tau = \gamma_0 G e^{-t/\lambda} \tag{2.38}$$

where $\lambda = \eta/G$ is called the *relaxation time*. The strain energy

Fig. 10. Kelvin model (*a*) and Maxwell model (*b*).

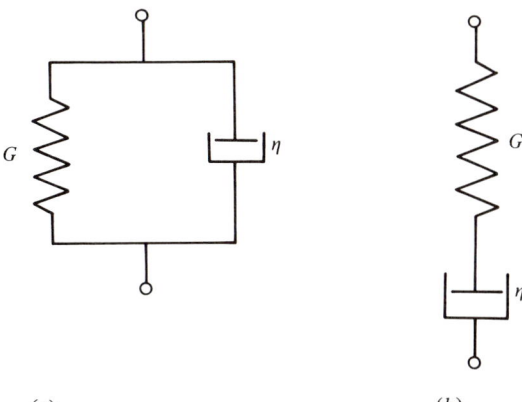

(a)   (b)

initially stored in the spring is dissipated in the dash pot, the mechanical energy being transformed into heat.

Equation (2.37) can be rewritten as

$$\dot{\gamma} = \frac{1}{G}\left(\frac{d\tau}{dt} + \frac{1}{\lambda}\tau\right) \tag{2.39}$$

If the deformation is very rapid, then the term τ/λ can be neglected, and by integrating we have $\gamma = \tau/G$. This indicates that the body behaves as a Hookean solid. If the deformation is very slow, then the term $d\tau/dt$ can be neglected, and we have $\dot{\gamma} = \tau/\eta$. This indicates that the body behaves as a Newtonian fluid.

Neither the Kelvin model nor the Maxwell model represent the behavior of real materials in normal situations. Thus, it is necessary to increase the number of springs and dash pots. A *four-element model* may be constructed from a Maxwell model in series with a Kelvin model.

(c) **Dynamic viscoelasticity**

Let us consider that the strain varies periodically:

$$\gamma = \gamma_0 \sin \omega t \tag{2.40}$$

where γ_0 is the amplitude of the strain, and ω is the angular frequency. In general, the stress is not in phase with the strain; it is written as

$$\tau = \tau_0 \sin(\omega t + \delta) \tag{2.41}$$

where τ_0 is the amplitude of the stress, and δ is the phase angle (Fig. 11(a)). It should be noted that the phase of the strain is always behind that of the stress.

Fig. 11. Dynamic modulus G' and loss modulus G''.

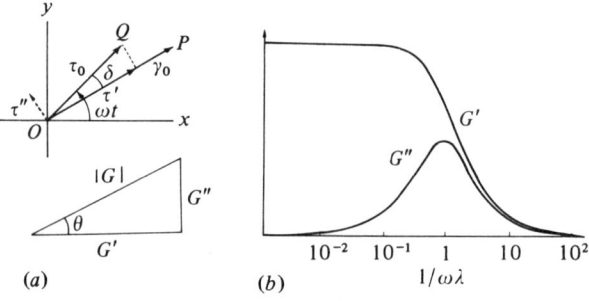

2.7 Viscoelasticity

Let us write Eq. (2.41) as

$$\tau = \tau_0 (\sin \omega t \cos \delta + \cos \omega t \sin \delta)$$

and put, for simplicity,

$$|G| = \tau_0/\gamma_0 \tag{2.42}$$

$$G' = |G| \cos \delta \tag{2.43}$$

$$G'' = |G| \sin \delta \tag{2.44}$$

Then we have

$$\tau = \tau_0 (G' \sin \omega t + G'' \cos \omega t) \tag{2.45}$$

In general, some of the mechanical energy is dissipated into heat. The energy dissipated in the body per unit volume in one cycle of oscillation is given by

$$w = \int \tau d\gamma = \int_0^{2\pi/\omega} \tau \frac{d\gamma}{dt} dt$$

or

$$w = \pi \gamma_0^2 G'' \tag{2.46}$$

If $\delta = 0$ or $\delta = \pi$, then $G'' = 0$, i.e. $w = 0$. Thus we see that G'' is proportional to the dissipated energy. The quantities $|G|$, G', and G'' are often called, respectively, the *absolute dynamic modulus*, the *dynamic modulus*, and the *loss modulus*. From Eqs. (2.43) and (2.44) we have

$$|G| = (G'^2 + G''^2)^{1/2} \tag{2.47}$$

$$\tan \delta = G''/G' \tag{2.48}$$

The relationship between $|G|$, G', G'', and δ is shown in Fig. 11(a).

In particular, the dynamic modulus and loss modulus of the Maxwell model can be obtained from Eq. (2.39) as follows:

$$G' = G \frac{\omega^2 \lambda^2}{1 + \omega^2 \lambda^2} \tag{2.49}$$

$$G'' = G \frac{\omega \lambda}{1 + \omega^2 \lambda^2} \tag{2.50}$$

Figure 11(b) shows the moduli G' and G'' as functions of frequency in the sinusoidal oscillation of a Maxwell model.

The strain γ and stress τ can be represented by vectors $\overrightarrow{OP}$ and $\overrightarrow{OQ}$, respectively. Let the components of the vectors $\overrightarrow{OQ}$ parallel and perpendicular to the direction OP be denoted by τ' and τ'', respectively, i.e.

$$\tau' = \tau_0 \cos \delta \qquad \tau'' = \tau_0 \sin \delta \qquad (2.51)$$

τ' is the component of the stress in phase with the strain, and τ'' 90° out of phase with the strain. From the relationships

$$G' = \frac{\tau_0}{\gamma_0} \cos \delta = \frac{\tau'}{\gamma_0} \qquad (2.52)$$

$$G'' = \frac{\tau_0}{\gamma_0} \sin \delta = \frac{\tau''}{\gamma_0} \qquad (2.53)$$

it is seen that G' is the ratio between τ' and γ_0, and G'' is the ratio between τ'' and γ_0. Instead of the two quantities G' and G'' let us introduce the following *complex modulus* for the sake of later chapters:

$$G^* = G' + iG'' \qquad (i^2 = -1) \qquad (2.54)$$

G' and G'' are, respectively, the real and imaginary part of the complex modulus.

Let us define the *complex viscosity* η^* by the relation

$$\eta^* = G^*/i\omega \qquad (2.55)$$

Then we have from Eq. (2.52)

$$\eta^* = \eta' - i\eta'' \qquad (2.56)$$

where

$$\eta' = G''/\omega \qquad \eta'' = G'/\omega \qquad (2.57)$$

and, in particular, η' is called the *dynamic viscosity*.

2.8 Strain energy density function

Let us consider a body subjected to a homogeneous deformation, i.e. all points in the body are in the same state of

2.8 Strain energy density function

strain. If we imagine a rectangular element of an appropriate orientation in the undeformed body, in the deformed body the element remains rectangular. Let the lengths of the sides of the element in the undeformed body be a, b, and c, and let these lengths become $\lambda_1 a$, $\lambda_2 b$, and $\lambda_3 c$ in the deformed body. Then λ_1, λ_2, and λ_3 are called the *principal extension ratios* (Fig. 12).

When a body is deformed elastically, work is done on the body by surface forces. This work is stored as strain energy. In order to avoid the complication of negative values, we consider that the strain energy is a function of λ_1^2, λ_2^2, and λ_3^2. The strain energy per unit volume, i.e. the strain energy density of the rectangular element as a function of λ_1^2, λ_2^2, and λ_3^2, is called the strain energy density function, W. It has been shown that W is a function of the three *strain invariants*:

$$\begin{aligned} I_1 &= \lambda_1^2 + \lambda_2^2 + \lambda_3^2 \\ I_2 &= \lambda_1^2 \lambda_2^2 + \lambda_2^2 \lambda_3^2 + \lambda_3^2 \lambda_1^2 \\ I_3 &= \lambda_1^2 \lambda_2^2 \lambda_3^2 \end{aligned} \qquad (2.58)$$

If the body is incompressible, I_3 is always equal to unity. Then we have

$$W = W(I_1, I_2) \qquad (2.59)$$

Fig. 12. Principal extension ratios $\lambda_1, \lambda_2, \lambda_3$.

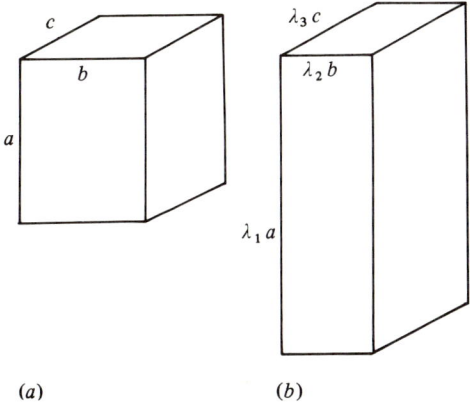

(a) (b)

with

$$I_1 = \lambda_1^2 + \lambda_2^2 + \frac{1}{\lambda_1^2 \lambda_2^2}$$
$$I_2 = \lambda_1^2 \lambda_2^2 + \frac{1}{\lambda_1^2} + \frac{1}{\lambda_2^2}$$
(2.60)

The strain energy density function enables us to obtain the stress in terms of λ_1 and λ_2 as follows:

$$\tau_1 - \tau_3 = \lambda_1 \frac{\partial W}{\partial \lambda_1} - \lambda_3 \frac{\partial W}{\partial \lambda_3}$$
$$\tau_2 - \tau_3 = \lambda_2 \frac{\partial W}{\partial \lambda_2} - \lambda_3 \frac{\partial W}{\partial \lambda_3}$$
$$\tau_1 - \tau_2 = \lambda_1 \frac{\partial W}{\partial \lambda_1} - \lambda_2 \frac{\partial W}{\partial \lambda_2}$$
(2.61)

It should be noted that τ_1, τ_2, and τ_3 cannot be determined uniquely, because $W(I_1, I_2)$ will never be influenced by an additive static hydrostatic pressure owing to the assumption of incompressibility.

According to the statistical theory of rubber elasticity, the strain energy density function of rubber is given by

$$W = nkT(I_1 - 3) \tag{2.62}$$

where n is the number of the network chains per unit volume, k is Boltzmann's constant, and T is the absolute temperature.

2.9 Thixotropy

A thixotropic gel is liquified by shaking or stirring, and sets again to a gel when at rest. Thixotropy is defined as an isothermal, reversible sol–gel transformation; this is now familiar to all workers in colloid science. Many colloidal systems do not exhibit thixotropy when pure, but most of them exhibit thixotropy when suitable concentrations of electrolytes or organic non-electrolytes are added.

Thixotropic fluids are a type of time-dependent non-Newtonian fluid; the apparent viscosity depends on the rate and duration of shear. Thixotropic fluids also possess a yield stress. This

2.9 Thixotropy

non-Newtonian behavior and thixotropy results from structural features of the fluids.

The flow curve of a thixotropic system produces a hysteresis loop in the shear stress–shear rate diagram when the shear rate steadily increases from zero to a maximum value and then immediately drops to zero. A thixotropic system also shows a torque–decay curve when the shear stress is plotted against the duration of the shear at a constant rate.

Thixotropy is important from the standpoint of hemorheology, because blood and protoplasm both display thixotropic behavior, as will be seen in Chapters 3 and 8.

3

Blood rheology

3.1 Blood

The ancient Greek philosopher Empedocles said: 'Blood is life.' The major task of blood is to supply oxygen to the tissues and to remove carbon dioxide via the lungs. In addition, blood supplies nutrients to the tissues, and removes non-gaseous metabolites. Many investigators have studied the complex role of blood in the cardiovascular systems of both man and animals, but there is still much to be learnt, despite modern sophisticated research.

The driving force for blood circulation is the heart, and the passages are the blood vessels. Flowing blood has peculiar rheological properties which are important in circulation physiology and clinical medicine.

Blood is divided into two main classes: formed elements, and continuous medium. The former consist of *red cells, white cells* and platelets, while the latter is *plasma*. The percentage volume of red cells is called the *hematocrit*, and is approximately 40–45%

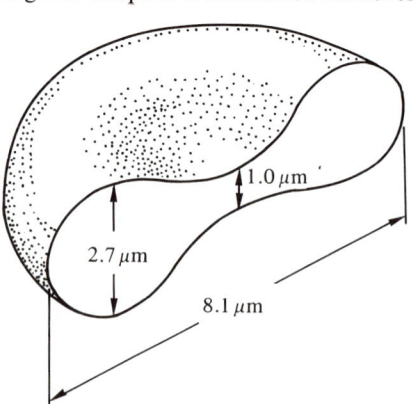

Fig. 13. Shape of a normal red cell at rest.

3.2 Aggregation of red cells

for an adult. Most of the formed elements are red cells, whose number density is approximately 5×10^6 mm^{-3}. The shape of a red cell is biconcave when at rest (Fig. 13). It is approximately 8 μm in diameter and 1 μm thick at the center.

Of the total volume of plasma, 90% is water, and 7% is proteins. Proteins in plasma consists of fibrinogen, globulin, albumin, and so on. Plasma from which fibrinogen is removed is called *serum*.

3.2   Aggregation of red cells

Red blood cells tend to pile up into rod-shaped formations, like a pile of coins, when at rest. These piles of cells are called *rouleaux*. Rouleaux can easily be observed in a drop of blood on glass under a light microscope. Human blood cells can form rouleaux, but practically no rouleaux are observed in bovine blood. However, horse cells show much more marked rouleaux formation than human cells.

In flowing blood, rouleaux are easily broken up and the cells are dispersed. Thus, in a healthy human no rouleaux can be observed in normal blood flow. But in some diseases red cells tend to aggregate intensely in flowing blood. (This occurs most frequently in infection.) This phenomenon is called *sludging*.

The cell aggregation and then rouleaux formation may be affected markedly by shear. Rouleaux can be formed or dispersed in slowly oscillating blood. In fact, King & Copley (1975) showed in an experiment that oscillatory motion greatly accelerates aggregation and rouleaux formation of human cells suspended in plasma at 0.01 Hz. Figure 14 is their photomicrograph for whole blood (44% hematocrit) in an oscillatory shear, in which the flow of red cells can be seen with the aid of a Weissenberg Rheogoniometer. Note that almost continuous rouleaux form and that there appears to be a gap between two cells in the rouleaux. The existence of the cell gap indicates that the rouleaux are unstable due to the oscillatory disturbance.

There are several factors which affect cell aggregation and rouleaux formation. The main factors are thought to be the reduction in the surface charge of the red cells, and the bridging between red cells by the long chain. Jan (1979) has emphasized the important role of macromolecular bridging between adjacent cell surfaces.

The bridging energy is a function of the nature of bridging and the sites between the macromolecule and the cell surface. Red cell aggregation may occur when the bridging force due to the surface adsorption of macromolecules overcomes both the electrostatic repulsive force and mechanical shearing force. Ultrastructural studies of cell aggregates show that intercellular distance is a function of macromolecular dimensions. On the other hand, the net aggre-

Fig. 14. Network of rouleaux formed at 0.01 Hz. (From King & Copley, 1975.)

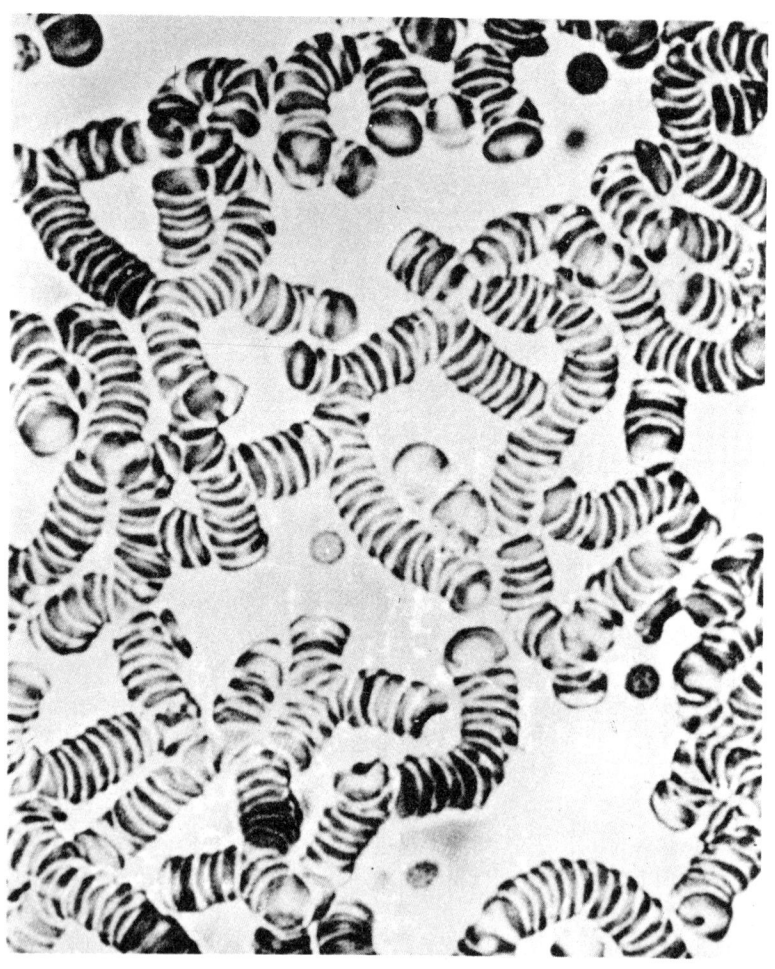

gation energy will be stored as a change in the membrane strain energy. Thus, the shape of cell aggregates may be determined by the net aggregation energy.

The addition of dextran to blood may affect cell aggregation and rouleaux formation by macromolecular bridging. According to Knox, Nordt, Seaman and Brooks (1977), dextran in excess of 40 000 molecular weight (MW) can induce weak cell aggregation of native human cells and formaldehyde-fixed cells, and this cell aggregation reaches maximum at a characteristic concentration of dextran.

Cell aggregation is usually measured by the microscopical method, the light intensity method, or the rheological method at low shear rates. A suitable method must be chosen to determine increases or decreases in cell aggregation. Sacks, Little & Kirk (1977) defined five classes of increasing aggregation on the basis of the variance in the light intensity. This procedure can produce an accurate measure of cell aggregation in both normal and diseased samples of blood under various conditions.

3.3 Sedimentation of red cells

The specific gravity of red cells is approximately 1.10, while that of plasma is 1.03. Thus red cells settle out of suspension under gravity because their density is greater than that of plasma. This phenomenon is called *sedimentation,* and the speed at which it occurs is often referred to as the *sedimentation rate.* An increased sedimentation rate for red cells is always regarded as abnormal, except in pregnancy.

Sedimentation is likely to occur *in vivo* in occluded blood vessels where flow is stagnant. Such sedimentation means that the viscosity of the blood will no longer be homogeneous. Little study has been made of how such sedimentation affects the blood flow *in vivo*.

When a red cell sinks through plasma, its speed will be influenced by many factors. *Stokes' law* states that the resistance to a rigid sphere moving through an infinite fluid is given by

$$D = 6\pi\mu a U \tag{3.1}$$

where D is the total force on the sphere, a is the radius of the sphere, U is the velocity of the sphere and μ is the viscosity of the fluid. The above law cannot be applied directly to a red cell falling through plasma, because its velocity is determined not only by the cell size, the densities of the cell and the plasma, and the viscosity of the plasma, but also by the cell shape and orientation. The aggregation of cells by clumping and rouleaux formation, and the interaction of these aggregates, will affect the sedimentation rate. Thus, a change in the sedimentation rate is a measure of change in the surface properties of the red cells, which is closely related to the cell aggregation.

The sedimentation rate is widely used to monitor the course of various diseases. In the sedimentation test, a long, narrow graduated tube is filled with citrated blood and the tube is kept vertical at a temperature of 22–27 °C. The upper level of the red cells and the height of the clear plasma column are usually recorded as the cells settle. Figure 15 shows a typical settling curve where the ordinate represents the length of the plasma column Y and the abscissa represents the time t. For convenience, the half time t_{50} is defined by the time for Y to attain $\frac{1}{2} Y_{t=\infty}$.

Several empirical attempts have been made to derive the settling curve. Puccini, Stasiw & Cerny (1977) offered a semi-empirical formula

$$Y(t) = \frac{Y_\infty}{1 + \exp\left[(\ln t - \ln t_{50})/b\right]} \tag{3.2}$$

where b is a positive constant. The curve Y/Y_∞ is expressed in terms of two parameters, b and t_{50}, and its shape is sigmoidal.

There are other clinical uses of the sedimentation rate. As mentioned in the previous section, oscillatory shear may disrupt the rouleaux network or promote contact between cells, affecting the

Fig. 15. Red cell sedimentation curve. (From Puccini *et al.* 1977.)

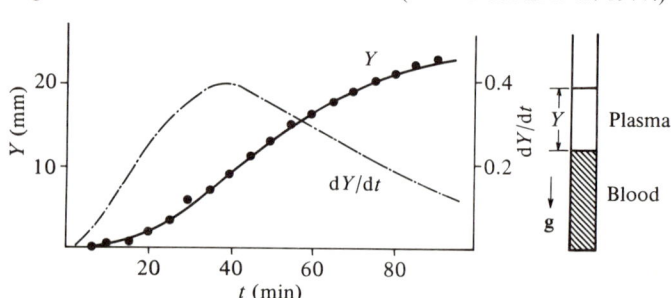

sedimentation process. Vincent & Oliver (1977) measured the sedimentation of washed red cells in dextran and/or saline solutions at controlled shear rates. The results obtained from these methods appear to be more reliable than those obtained from conventional vertical settling tubes. Their methods may be useful for clinical sedimentation tests because of their speed and reliability.

3.4 Non-Newtonian viscosity

The viscosity of human blood can be measured by the shear rate, using a cone–plate viscometer or a coaxial rotating cylinder viscometer. Whole blood is non-Newtonian and shear-thinning. Figure 16 shows the apparent viscosity of human blood as a function of the shear rate (Wells, Merrill & Gabelnick, 1962). The apparent viscosity of whole blood increases very rapidly with decreasing shear rate. Red cell suspension in saline solution is also non-Newtonian, but its absolute value of viscosity is lower than that of whole blood. Plasma appears to exhibit Newtonian viscosity in Fig. 15. It should be noted that some authors describe plasma as non-Newtonian, emphasizing the influence of fibrinogen on its behavior. Plasma is known to exhibit a unique relaxation phenomenon. In fact, stress induced in plasma by suddenly applied shear may gradually decrease to zero. This suggests a weak network

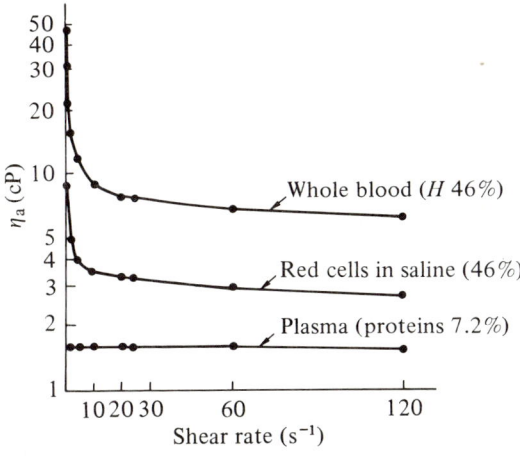

Fig. 16. Apparent viscosity of blood vs. shear rate. (From Wells et al. 1962.)

structure of fibrinogen which can be broken under a small shear stress. The fibrinogen may be responsible for plasma rheology, but there is no conclusive evidence about whether plasma is non-Newtonian or not.

The non-Newtonian behavior of blood and red cell suspensions in saline solution is closely related to the existence of red cells. It is generally considered that a cause of the non-Newtonian behavior lies in the reversible breakdown of aggregates, rouleaux, or some weak bonds between red cells with increasing shear rate. At present, little is known about the molecular structure of the weak bonds, but in blood it is certain that weak bonds between red cells may be formed through proteins, particularly fibrinogen. Red cell suspension in saline solution does not include any protein, so there can be only a physical association between red cells.

Another cause of the non-Newtonian behavior of blood is thought to be the deformation and orientation of red cells in the blood flow. The deformation of red cells in response to shear stress makes possible an alignment of their major axes with flow, with a consequent reduction of viscosity. (We will look at this in more detail in Chapter 4.) This mechanism of cell deformation and orientation may be most effective at high shear rates. Schmid-Schönbein (1977) states that in the non-Newtonian viscosity of blood, or red cell suspension in saline solution, cell aggregation is predominant at low shear stress (below $1 \, \text{dyn} \, \text{cm}^{-2}$), but cell deformation and orientation are effective at high shear stress (above $10 \, \text{dyn} \, \text{cm}^{-2}$).

3.5 Thixotropy and viscoelasticity

As can be seen from the torque–decay curve or a hysteresis loop of a sample of whole blood, using a Weissenberg Rheogoniometer (Fig. 17), whole human blood exhibits time-dependent rheological behavior. More strictly, it complies with thixotropy as defined in Chapter 2. The time-dependent rheological behavior of blood and thixotropy may be closely related to the progressive change in the internal structure of blood. Copley *et al.* (1975) and Usami *et al.* (1975) demonstrated how rouleaux are broken down or formed during shearing, and offered a rheological equation to describe the thixotropy of whole blood using a model of isothermal structural change induced by a shear stress.

3.5 Thixotropy and viscoelasticity

Blood exhibits viscoelastic properties. Thurston (1973) studied the viscoelastic behavior of blood in oscillatory flow through a tube, and determined the frequency dependence of the viscosity and elasticity of blood and plasma in the range from 0.03 to 50 Hz (Fig. 18). In blood, the elastic component of the viscosity, η'', is of appreciable magnitude at all the frequencies measured. This indicates that under these conditions blood should be regarded as a viscoelastic fluid. In plasma, the viscosity component is independent

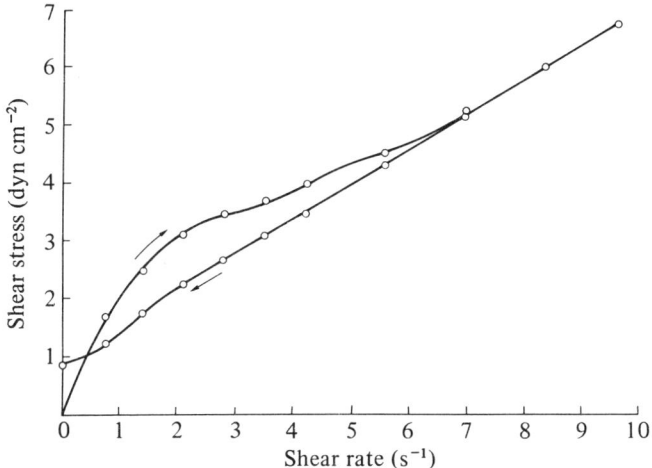

Fig. 17. Shear stress vs. shear rate for blood. (From Huang et al., 1975.)

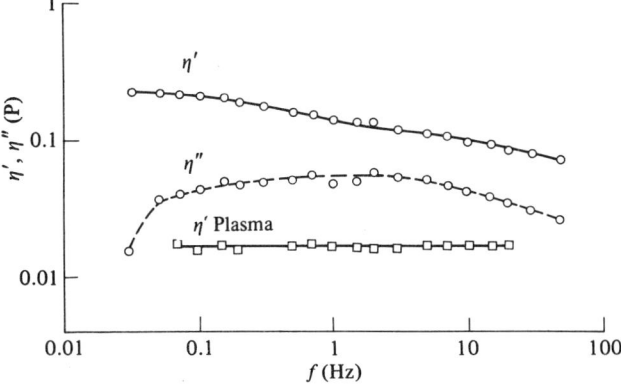

Fig. 18. Frequency dependence of the complex viscosity. (From Thurston, 1973.)

of frequency in this range. Thus plasma shows no measurable elastic behavior.

The oscillatory test is normally used for measuring the viscoelasticity of blood and red cell suspension in plasma or Ringer solution. The measured dynamic modulus G' provides an indication of the elastic modulus of the cells (presumably that of the cell membrane). Markedly increasing G' for red cell suspension in plasma may reflect the elastic behavior of the rouleaux formed by red cells. Decreasing G' may indicate some disturbances in rouleaux size and deformation. Chien et al. (1966) investigated the viscoelastic behavior of normal human blood over a lower frequency range in cone–plate geometry. At the hematocrit of 45%, the non-dispersed suspension of red cells in Ringer solution shows a normal value in G', but the rouleaux formed in the presence of the aggregating plasma proteins show a six-fold increase in G'. Their finding is supplemented by the results of Copley et al. and Usami et al. According to their microscopic studies, at low frequencies of oscillation (near 0.01 Hz) suspensions of red cells in plasma show extensive rouleaux formation over an extensive period of time, and these large rouleaux undergo cyclic elastic distortion at the imposed frequency. The rouleaux size becomes progressively smaller as the oscillation frequency increases from about 0.1 Hz. These observations correspond well to the fact that the value of G' rises in the low-frequency range and decreases with the increase in the oscillation frequency at about 0.1 Hz. Thus it appears that the change in the value of G' may be due to rouleaux formation disturbed by oscillatory shear.

Rheological behavior of blood in various transient flows may be a consequence of the internal organization, which in turn depends on red cell aggregation and rouleaux formation. Healy & Joly (1975) studied the transient response to shear stress at very low shear rates ($\dot{\gamma}$ of $10^{-2} - 10^{-1}$ s^{-1}) where thixotropy effects appear, and elucidated the role of shear stress in the transient flow from a three-dimensional network structure in blood at rest. The phenomena observed in the transient response to shear stress were classified into the following: (i) When the applied shear stress is high enough to break down the network structure in blood, the apparent viscosity of blood immediately falls until blood behaves

3.5 Thixotropy and viscoelasticity

like a Newtonian liquid. (ii) When the shear stress is so low that some time must lapse before the network structure breaks down, the apparent viscosity of blood decreases until it reaches a stationary value in a few seconds.

In order to predict the transient rheological behavior of blood, it is sometimes necessary to construct the complete equation governing blood flow. To this end, a number of constitutive equations for blood flow have been proposed by many investigators. Huang et al. (1975) proposed a viscoelastic equation as a model for blood, which originates from the first author's study of blood under thermodynamic considerations. Phillips & Deutsch (1975) introduced a *nonlinear viscoelastic model* for blood. Their model includes a normal stress term that has not been taken into consideration in most rheological models of blood. The validity of the model was tested by applying it to two typical flow problems: two-dimensional channel flow, and circular Couette flow. In the channel flow, the velocity profile was predicted to be more blunt than parabolic. In the Couette viscometric flow, a stress overshoot was predictable from the normal stress term. It is interesting to note that their model does not need to assume a cell-free layer by which the stress overshoot phenomenon has been explained. It is known that normal stress effects occur in various viscoelastic fluids, including blood, but there is no experiment to evaluate to what extent normal stress can influence blood flow.

Some attempts have been made to unify all the rheological properties of blood, such as non-Newtonian viscosity, viscoelasticity, and thixotropy. Thurston (1979) proposed a unifying hypothesis, introducing a new concept of rheological equilibrium and non-equilibrium to distinguish between non-equilibrium thixotropy and equilibrium viscosity and viscoelasticity. Two characteristic periods were considered: the relaxation time, which is of primary importance in assessing the equilibrium properties for the viscosity and viscoelasticity, and the characteristic time of the rate of breakdown and recovery of the internal structures, which is central to assessing the non-equilibrium thixotropic properties. The degradation function and the general Maxwell model have been used for the analysis of non-Newtonian viscosity and nonlinear viscoelasticity.

3.6 Factors affecting blood viscosity

The viscosity of blood and red cell suspensions is affected by several factors, such as hematocrit, the plasma proteins, red cell deformation, aggregation, and so on.

(a) Hematocrit

Hematocrit is the major factor affecting the viscosity of whole blood and red cell suspensions in saline solution. The viscosity of whole blood increases as hematocrit rises.

The viscosity of a red cell suspension in saline solution also increases as hematocrit rises. Plasma with a small volume fraction of red cells behaves like a Newtonian fluid. The viscosity of such suspensions may be expressed approximately by the equation:

$$\frac{\eta}{\eta_p} = \frac{1}{1 - \alpha \phi} \qquad (3.3)$$

where η_p is the plasma viscosity, α is a constant related to the shape of suspended particles, and ϕ is the volume fraction. The above equation holds very well up to $\phi = 0.05$. Charm & Kurland (1972) showed that it is valid up to $\phi = 0.6$ if α is calculated from the equation:

$$\alpha = 0.076 \exp\left[2.49\phi + \frac{1107}{T} \exp(-1.69\phi)\right] \qquad (3.4)$$

where T is the absolute temperature.

(b) Plasma proteins

The viscosity of plasma is determined primarily by the concentration of proteins present, especially fibrinogen. In a healthy adult, the concentrations of various plasma proteins remain surprisingly constant. For this reason, close examination of their concentrations is used in the diagnosis of various diseases.

Globulin concentration increases in diseases. Especially, the α-globulins increase following injury, an operation, or acute infection; γ-globulins increase following infections, and new globulin-type proteins are formed in myeloma and macroglobulinemia. Fibrinogen also increases in some diseases. Moreover, increases in globulin concentration are often accompanied by decreases in albumin concentration. Though plasma viscosity is closely related to the concentrations of different proteins, it is difficult to diagnose diseases simply by measuring plasma viscosity.

(c) *Red cell deformation*

Red cells may affect the viscosity of whole blood and cell suspensions in saline solution, changing their hydrodynamic effective volume in the shear flow. The deformation of red cells is influenced by many factors, such as the elasticity and viscosity of red cells, the internal viscosity of cells, the size and shape of cells, ATP content, the osmotic pressure of blood, the oxygen pressure, and so on. These will be discussed in detail in Chapter 4, but we consider here *Dintenfass's equation* (Dintenfass, 1975) for blood viscosity, which includes the effects of red cell deformation:

$$\eta_r = (1 - CkT)^{-2.5} \tag{3.5}$$

Here η_r is the relative viscosity defined by η/η_p, C is the volume concentration of red cells, k is the packing coefficient of red cells, including the effect of plasma trapping, and T is the Taylor factor defined in Chapter 2. In his calculation of the internal viscosity of red cells, the term Ck is replaced by the microhematocrit, H, as an approximation. Then, the Taylor factor T can be obtained from Eq. (2.33) in the form: $T = (1 - \eta_r^{-0.4})/H$. The ratio of the *internal viscosity* of red cells to that of plasma, p, is calculated in terms of T as follows: $p = (T - 0.4)/(1 - T)$. Then the internal viscosity of red cells can be calculated in terms of H and η_r. Dintenfass (1975) applied his blood viscosity equation to diagnosis of various diseases, such as renal failure, hemodialysis, kidney transplantation, cancer, and so on. Since his equation for blood viscosity includes some arbitrary assumptions about red cell rheology, it must be used with caution.

Let us now consider the cone–plate viscometer, which is often used to measure the apparent viscosity of blood and cell suspensions. In this type of viscometer, the controlled shear rate in the flow field is assumed to be constant under the following conditions: (i) the angle between cone and plate is very small (approximately one half of a degree), (ii) the flow is so slow that convection is negligible. It must be emphasized that the second condition is no longer satisfied for shear stresses of the order of 100 dyn cm^{-2} or more. In the high rotational flow, red cells will be subjected to a force which produces a shift in the radial direction. In fact, Heuser (1978) calculated the radial pressure distribution and the flow structure in the high rotational flow of Newtonian fluids. There is good agreement between theoretical and experimental results for Newtonian fluids, but not for blood. A shift in red cell concentration was detected in the radial direction. This indicates that the viscosity of blood measured with the cone–plate viscometer must be checked in the shear stress range.

3.7 Casson fluid

(a) Casson's equation

Casson (1959) used a cone–plate viscometer to study flow properties of varnishes filled with pigments, and found an empirical relationship between the shear stress, τ, and the shear rate, $\dot{\gamma}$, as follows:

$$\tau^{1/2} = k_0 + k_1 \dot{\gamma}^{1/2} \tag{3.6}$$

where k_0 and k_1 are positive constants whose values depend on the properties of suspensions. The relation (3.6) is called *Casson's equation*. Later that year (1959), Scott Blair plotted $\tau^{1/2}$ against $\dot{\gamma}^{1/2}$ for whole blood, plasma, and serums of several species; he showed that they produced excellent straight lines, and also that they

Fig. 19. Casson plot for human blood. (From Scott Blair, 1959.)

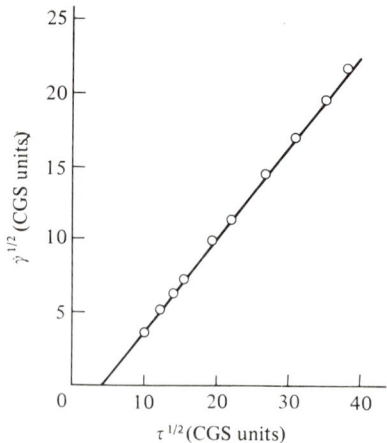

3.7 Casson fluid

extrapolated to the origin only for Newtonian fluids (Fig. 19).

If we put $k_1 = \eta_C^{1/2}$ and $k_0 = f_C^{1/2}$, we can rewrite the above Casson relation as follows:

$$\dot{\gamma} = (1/\eta_C)(\tau^{1/2} - f_C^{1/2})^2 \tag{3.7}$$

In the above, η_C is measured in units of viscosity while f_C is in units of stress; thus η_C and f_C are called the *Casson viscosity* and the *Casson yield stress*, respectively. The plot of $\dot{\gamma}^{1/2}$ against $\tau^{1/2}$ gives a straight line which intersects with the abscissa at the point $\tau = f_C$. This line is usually called the *Casson plot*.

Casson's equation may provide a good description of the rheological behavior of whole blood. If the angle between the Casson plot and the abscissa is θ, the Casson viscosity is determined from the angle θ as follows:

$$\eta_C = 1/\tan^2 \theta \tag{3.8}$$

Various empirical formulas have been proposed for the relationship between the apparent viscosity of blood, η_a, and the hematocrit. An empirical formula has recently been proposed by Shiga *et al.* (1979) as follows:

$$\ln(\eta_C/\eta_p) = \text{const } H \tag{3.9}$$

where η_p is the plasma viscosity and H is the hematocrit.

Casson derived his own equation theoretically, making certain assumptions. He assumed that flocculated particles in a suspension form chain-like groups through mutual attraction, and that the viscosity of the suspension may be governed by the size of the groups. According to his theory, when the suspension flows, the chain-like groups are subjected to destructive stresses with the magnitude dependent upon the shear rate and the size of a group. Consequently, the equilibrium group size, and hence the viscosity, may vary with the shear rate. For simplicity, he treated the groups as long cylindrical rods of axial ratio J, defined by the ratio of length to width, and assumed a relationship between the axial ratio and the shear rate in the form: $J = a + b/(\eta_0 \dot{\gamma})^{1/2}$, where η_0 is the viscosity of the suspending medium and a, b are positive constants. Making some arbitrary assumptions, he succeeded in deriving Eq. (3.6).

From the standpoint of Casson's idea, Murata (1976) explained non-Newtonian behavior of blood at very low shear rates in a more sophisticated way by applying the theory of coagulation in colloids to the process of rouleaux formation. The expression for the average size of rouleaux in dynamic equilibrium was constructed so that it could be reduced to Casson's assumptions about the size of rouleaux and shear rate. The shear stress–shear rate relationship obtained for a dilute suspension of red cells showed that the plot of square root of shear rate vs. the square root of shear stress lies on the curve whose asymptote is given by Casson's equation.

Casson's concept of the non-Newtonian mechanism in suspensions is based on the formation of chain-like groups of suspended particles. As mentioned previously, Casson's equation holds for human blood as well as bovine blood. Since bovine blood does not form rouleaux, Casson's idea will not be valid for all blood. Thus, quite a different theory is needed to explain Casson's equation for blood.

A unified theory of the constitutive equations for non-Newtonian suspensions was developed by the present writer. He assumed, after Scott Blair, that the bonds formed between suspended particles were broken down gradually with increasing shear stress or shear rate. Based on this suspension model, the differential equation for the flow curve of suspension was derived in the form (Oka, 1971):

$$\frac{d\tau}{(\tau + C_1)\alpha} = k_1 \frac{d\dot{\gamma}}{(\dot{\gamma} + C_2)\alpha} \tag{3.10}$$

where k_1, C_1, C_2 are constants and α is a dimensionless parameter ($\alpha \leqq 1$). In the above, making $C_1 = C_2 = 0$ and $\alpha = \frac{1}{2}$, we have Casson's equation. Thus, the above equation includes Casson's equation as a special case. In addition, the present derivation dispenses with Casson's assumption of the formation of long cylindrical rods. For these reasons, the present unified theory covers bovine blood as well as human blood.

(b) Casson yield stress

It is extremely difficult to measure shear stress and shear rate when the shear rate is very low. But it is generally accepted that blood will not flow unless the shear stress exceeds the Casson

3.7 Casson fluid

yield stress. The yield stress is governed by factors such as hematocrit, fibrinogen concentration, and so on.

Merrill et al. (1963) found that blood exhibited no yield stress at hematocrits below a certain critical value, H_c. At hematocrits exceeding H_c, the yield stress was given by:

$$f_C^{1/3} = (A/100)(H - H_c) \tag{3.11}$$

where $A = (0.008 \text{ dyn cm}^{-2})^{1/3}$, $H_c = 5\text{–}8\%$.

Red cell suspension in saline solution may also exhibit yield stress, provided that the hematocrit is sufficiently high. Merrill, Margetts, Cokelet, & Gilliland (1965) found that the fibrinogen added to red cell suspension in saline solution produces increased aggregation, and that the yield stress increases with increasing concentration as follows:

$$f_C^{1/2} = 0.36B\left(\frac{1}{1-\phi} - 1\right) \tag{3.12}$$

where B is a function of fibrinogen concentration and ϕ is the volume fraction of red cells. Red cell suspension in serum without fibrinogen may also possess a small but definite yield stress. Chien et al. (1966) showed that the yield stress for red cell suspension in serum is approximately half that for red cell suspension in plasma. Furthermore, at sufficiently high concentrations, red cell suspension in saline solution is found to possess a yield stress smaller than that in plasma (Chien et al., 1966). Copley, Luchini & Whelan (1967) found that minute amounts of fibrinogen–fibrin complex can lead to dramatic increases in the yield stress.

The detailed mechanism of the yield stress is not yet known; but it is known that direct contact of red cells with each other, and aggregates of red cells with fibrinogen, are responsible for the yield stress. Fibrinogen is a rod-like molecule containing three spheres. One end of a fibrinogen molecule may be adsorbed in the membrane of a red cell, and the other end may be adsorbed in the membrane of another red cell, i.e. a weak network structure may be formed of red cells and fibrinogen molecules.

The yield stress for human blood has usually been measured under quasi-static conditions. Walburn & Schneck (1976) cast some doubt on whether yield stress exists at all when blood is flowing.

Further, there is some doubt about whether yield stress really does affect the blood flow *in vivo* or not. Bate (1977) suggested that the yield stress and viscosity of blood may vary in low shear flow through tubes, probably due to a structural effect of orientation or interaction of cells. Since the yield stress is extremely small, and moreover decreases with shear rate, the yield stress will not have an important effect on blood flow *in vivo*. It should be noted that the addition of an anti-coagulant may reduce or eliminate the interactions between fibrinogen and red cells which cause the yield stress.

(c) Steady flow in a cylindrical tube

Let us consider the steady flow of a fluid obeying Casson's equation through a straight cylindrical tube of uniform radius R and of length L under the pressure difference Δp. The following assumptions are made regarding the motion of the fluid: (i) the fluid is incompressible; (ii) fluid flow is laminar; (iii) the flow is parallel to the axis of the tube; (iv) the flow is steady; (v) there is no slip at the wall.

The rheological behavior of the Casson fluid is specified by the flow curve:

$$\left. \begin{aligned} f(\tau) &= \frac{1}{\eta_C}(\sqrt{\tau} - \sqrt{f_C})^2 & (\tau > f_C) \\ &= 0 & (\tau < f_C) \end{aligned} \right\} \quad (3.13)$$

where η_C is the Casson viscosity and f_C is the Casson yield stress. Substitution of Eq. (3.13) into Eq. (2.17) yields the velocity distribution (Oka, 1965):

$$\left. \begin{aligned} u &= \frac{\Delta p}{4\eta_C L}[R^2 - r^2 - \tfrac{8}{3}r_C^{1/2}(R^{3/2} - r^{3/2}) \\ &\quad + 2r_C(R-r)] & (r > r_C) \\ &= \frac{\Delta p}{4\eta_C L}(\sqrt{R} - \sqrt{r_C})^3(\sqrt{R} + \tfrac{1}{3}\sqrt{r_C}) & (r < r_C) \end{aligned} \right\} \quad (3.14)$$

where r_C is defined by:

$$f_C = (\Delta p/2L)r_C \quad (3.15)$$

3.7 Casson fluid

r_C is the value of r at which the shear stress becomes equal to f_C. Let us further introduce a critical pressure difference p_C defined by the relation:

$$f_C = (p_C/2L)R \qquad (3.16)$$

p_C being the pressure difference for which the shear stress at the wall becomes equal to the yield value f_C. Then Eq. (3.14) corresponds to $\Delta p > p_C$. When $\Delta p < p_C$, we have $u = 0$. From the above relations, the velocity profile is shown schematically in Fig. 20.

We now consider the flow rate. Substitution of Eq. (3.13) into

Fig. 20. Velocity profile of a Casson fluid in a tube.

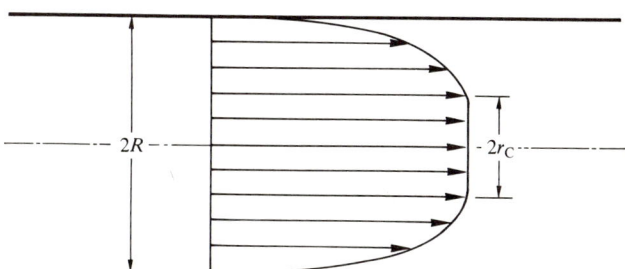

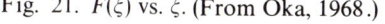

Fig. 21. $F(\xi)$ vs. ξ. (From Oka, 1968.)

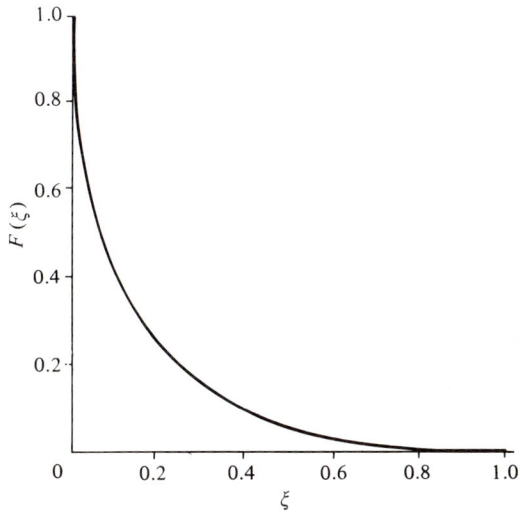

Eq. (2.18) yields

$$Q = \frac{\pi R^4}{8\eta_C L}\left[\Delta p - \frac{16}{7}\sqrt{p_C}\sqrt{\Delta p} + \frac{4}{3}p_C - \frac{1}{21}\frac{p_C^4}{\Delta p^3}\right] \quad (\Delta p > p_C)$$
$$= 0 \quad (\Delta p < p_C)$$
(3.17)

The pressure–flow curve touches the abscissa at the point $\Delta p = p_C$. Equation (3.17) can be rewritten as

$$Q = \frac{\pi R^4}{8\eta_C}\frac{\Delta p}{L}F(\xi) \tag{3.18}$$

where

$$F(\xi) = 1 - \frac{16}{7}\sqrt{\xi} + \frac{4}{3}\xi - \frac{1}{21}\xi^4 \tag{3.19}$$

and ξ is a dimensionless quantity defined by

$$\xi = p_C/\Delta p \tag{3.20}$$

$F(\xi)$ is plotted against ξ in Fig. 21. In the limiting case when $f_C \to 0$, i.e. $\xi \to 0$, Eq. (3.18) becomes Poiseuille's law, as would be expected.

It should be noted that the increase in flow rate with increasing radius arises not only from the term R^4, but also from the term $\xi = 2Lf_C/R\Delta p$, where ξ decreases. While $F(\xi)$ was first formulated by the present writer, the same expression was arrived at independently by several later investigators.

3.8 Plasma layer

(a) A general description

A cell-free marginal zone is formed in blood flow through small blood vessels as well as small glass tubes. The cell-free zone consists mainly of plasma; this zone is usually called the *plasma layer*, while the remainder is called the *central core*.

The existence of the plasma layer in arterioles, venules and capillaries in various species of living animals, as well as in small glass tubes, has long been known. Apparently, Haller and Spallanzani knew of it in the 18th century. Poiseuille (1836) noted that the plasma layer increased as the flow rate increased.

3.8 Plasma layer

There is no plasma layer in blood at rest. How is the plasma layer related to the blood flow? In order to examine the relationship between the thickness of plasma layer and the flow rate, Taylor (1955) and Bayliss (1959) measured the transmissivity of light in flows of red cell suspensions in saline solution through small glass tubes using a microphotometer. The transmissivity measured in the direction perpendicular to the axis of the tube increased with increasing mean velocity of the suspension. Their finding indicates that the thickness of plasma layer increases with the mean velocity, but that a part of the increase may be due to the orientation of red cells in flows. Later, Charm, Kurland & Brown (1968) showed that the thickness of the plasma layer does not change with the mean velocity in a sufficiently fast flow. Bayliss (1952) demonstrated the presence of similar phenomena in defibrinated dog blood.

(b) Effect of the plasma layer on the pressure–flow relationship

We shall consider from a theoretical standpoint the effect of the plasma layer on the pressure–flow relationship of blood in narrow tubes. Since this relationship depends, of course, upon the rheological properties of the central core, we consider two cases: where the central core is regarded as a Bingham body, and as a Casson fluid.

Let us denote the inner radius of the tube by R, and the thickness of the plasma layer by δ. Then, the radius of the central core is given by

$$R_c = \gamma R \tag{3.21}$$

with

$$\gamma = 1 - (\delta/R) \tag{3.22}$$

(i) Case where the central core is regarded as a Bingham body.

Let us denote the Bingham yield stress and the Bingham viscosity by f_B and η_B, respectively. Then the flow curve for the Bingham body is generally expressed in the form:

$$\left.\begin{aligned} f(\tau) &= \frac{1}{\eta_B}(\tau - f_B) & (\tau > f_B) \\ &= 0 & (\tau < f_B) \end{aligned}\right\} \tag{3.23}$$

In this case the flow rate is given by

$$Q = \frac{\pi R^4}{8}\frac{\Delta p}{L}\left[\frac{1}{\eta_B}\left(\gamma^4 - \frac{4}{3}\gamma^3\xi + \frac{1}{3}\xi^4\right)\right.$$
$$\left.+\frac{1}{\eta_p}(1-\gamma^4)\right] \qquad \left(\Delta p > \frac{p_B}{\gamma}\right)$$
$$= \frac{\pi R^4}{8\eta_p}\frac{\Delta p}{L}(1-\gamma^4) \qquad \left(\Delta p < \frac{p_B}{\gamma}\right) \qquad (3.24)$$

with

$$\xi = p_B/\Delta p \qquad (3.25)$$

p_B is defined by

$$f_B = (p_B/2L)R \qquad (3.26)$$

This is the pressure difference at which the shear stress at the wall becomes equal to f_B.

(ii) Case where the central core is regarded as a Casson fluid.

Let us denote the Casson yield stress and the Casson viscosity by f_C and η_C, respectively, and let p_C be defined by

$$f_C = (p_C/2L)R \qquad (3.27)$$

p_C being the pressure difference at which the shear stress at the wall becomes equal to f_C. In this case the flow rate is given by:

$$Q = \frac{\pi R^4}{8}\frac{\Delta p}{L}\left[\frac{1}{\eta_C}\left(\gamma^4 - \frac{16}{7}\gamma^{7/2}\xi^{1/2} + \frac{4}{3}\gamma^3\xi - \frac{1}{21}\xi^4\right)\right.$$
$$\left.+\frac{1}{\eta_p}(1-\gamma^4)\right] \qquad \left(\Delta p > \frac{p_C}{\gamma}\right)$$
$$= \frac{\pi R^4}{8}\frac{\Delta p}{L}(1-\gamma^4) \qquad \left(\Delta p < \frac{p_C}{\gamma}\right) \qquad (3.28)$$

3.9 Radial migration

The presence of plasma layer in blood flow through a narrow tube suggests that red cells near the wall are affected by some force towards the axis of tube so that they are carried towards the central region. The transference of red cells is referred to as *radial migration* or *axial accumulation*.

In recent years, many studies of radial migration have been

3.9 Radial migration

described by Mason, Goldsmith, Segré, Silberberg, and so on (Goldsmith & Mason, 1965, Segré & Silberberg, 1962). Most of the studies can be put in the category of fluid mechanics. Below, we describe their main experimental and theoretical results.

In studies of the underlying mechanism controlling the radial migration of red cells, it is most convenient to consider the behavior of a single model particle in a flow through a small tube. As a model of a red cell, a small rigid sphere of the same density as the fluid carrying it has often been employed. Sometimes a rigid disc or rod with a shape similar to that of red cells is used. Sometimes a flexible or deformable disc or rod, or a drop of fluid, is used to simulate the effect of the deformation of red cells. In each case the model particle is placed in a Poiseuille flow through a long straight tube. A very slow, or slow, flow is maintained.

The experimental results are generally as follows. If the Poiseuille flow is very slow, a rigid particle (sphere, disc or rod) does not exhibit radial migration at all; but a flexible disc, rod or deformable drop does exhibit radial migration, and reaches an equilibrium position on the tube axis. However, at very high flow rate, a rigid particle initially near the wall moves towards the axis of the tube, but a rigid particle near the axis moves towards the wall. Eventually, rigid particles move towards an equilibrium position about $0.6R$ from the axis (R being the tube radius). This phenomenon is called the *tubular pinch effect* or *Segré–Silberberg effect*. However a deformable drop shows radial migration at all speeds.

Theoretical studies using the linearized Navier–Stokes equation predict no migration with a rigid sphere. On the other hand, the full Navier–Stokes equation involving convective terms predicts a force on a rigid sphere in the radial direction. But the predicted force is insufficient to explain the Segré–Silberberg effect.

A rigid particle is known to rotate in a Poiseuille flow. In particular, a sphere rotates at a constant angular velocity, but a disc or rod does not maintain a constant angular velocity. From observation of particle rotation, the Magnus effect has been suggested as a mechanism underlying radial migration. But the Magnus force driving a particle away from the tube wall is known to be extremely small in the case of a red cell, because of the very small relative velocity of the particle to the neighboring fluid.

It is probable that the radial migration of red cells is due to the deformation of red cells in a Poiseuille flow. In order to clarify the effect of deformation of red cells on the axial drift, Palmer & Betts (1975) used fresh and aldehyde-hardened red cells. The axial drift of the two kinds was determined in flows through 25 μm capillary slits by measuring the packed-cell volume in effluents from five terminal slit branches (Fig. 22). With both fresh and hardened cells, the axial drift increased progressively as slit length

Fig. 22. Flow in a branching slit apparatus. (From Palmer & Betts, 1975.)

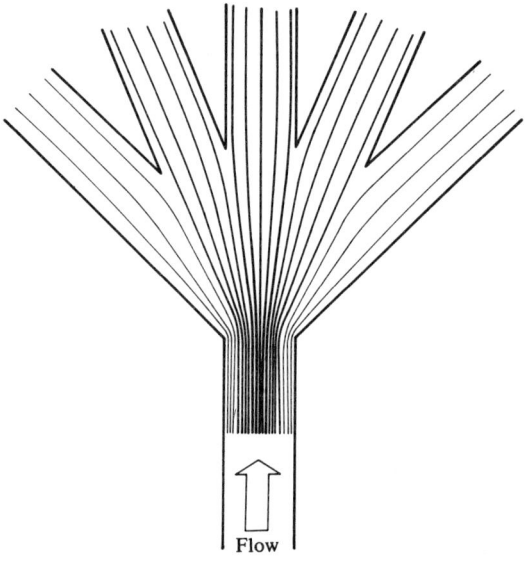

Fig. 23. Redistribution of suspended particles in a constricted tube. (From Whitmore, 1959.)

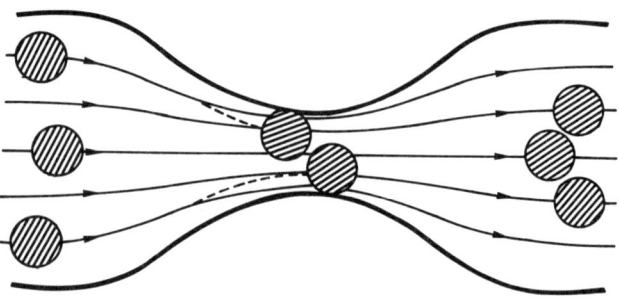

was increased from 0.5 to 5 mm. At a length of slit (0.5 mm) similar to that found in physiology, the axial drift had already reached half the final value it reaches at 10 mm. Furthermore, the fresh cells drifted much more than the hardened cells. Their findings strongly suggest that the deformation of red cells plays an essential role in radial migration.

A number of different mechanisms have been proposed to explain the presence of the plasma layer. Let us consider one mechanism causing this cell-free layer, suggested by Maude & Whitmore (1958). With blood flow in a constricted and small tube, near the point of the construction red cells in the converging streamlines which pass through the constriction very close to the wall should undergo slight radial displacement (Fig. 23). At the end of the constriction, the red cells would follow diverging streamlines so that peripheral cells would not necessarily return to their original radial portion. This mechanism is of great interest in explaining the presence of a plasma zone near an obstacle; but it is necessary to take into account that while red cells at rest are discoid, they can deform easily in shear flows.

3.10 Flow of red cell suspensions in small tubes

(a) Pressure–flow relationship

Let us first study the relationship between pressure and flow of red cell suspensions. Figure 24 shows the pressure–flow curves for red cells suspended in acid–citrate–dextrose (ACD) in a glass tube of 472 μm for a variety of hematocrits at 25.5 °C (Haynes & Burton, 1959). All the pressure–flow curves pass through the origin in such a way that the flow rate increases as the pressure gradient increases; the curves are strongly nonlinear at low pressure gradients but nearly linear at high pressure gradients. The back extrapolations of their linear segments appear to converge at a common point on the negative flow-axis. All the pressure–flow curves may then be approximated by the equation:

$$Q = M(R, H)P - B(R)[1 - \exp(-k(R, H))P] \qquad (3.29)$$

In the above, Q is the flow rate and P is the pressure gradient. $M(R, H)$ represents the slope of the linear segments of curves, depending on the tube radius R and on the hematocrit H. $B(R)$

represents the back extrapolation on the negative flow-axis, depending only on the tube radius, $k(R, H)$ represents an exponential constant to be determined by the shape of the non-linear part of curves. Haynes & Burton (1959) found that the back extrapolation B could be expressed in terms of R in the form:

$$\log B = 3 \log R + \text{const} \tag{3.30}$$

Gordon (1970) put forward a modified marginal zone theory in order to explain the experimental findings by Haynes. Here we re-examine this problem under the assumption that the central core in blood flow is a Bingham body. Then the pressure–flow curve from Eq.(3.24) for blood flow through a rigid tube of radius R

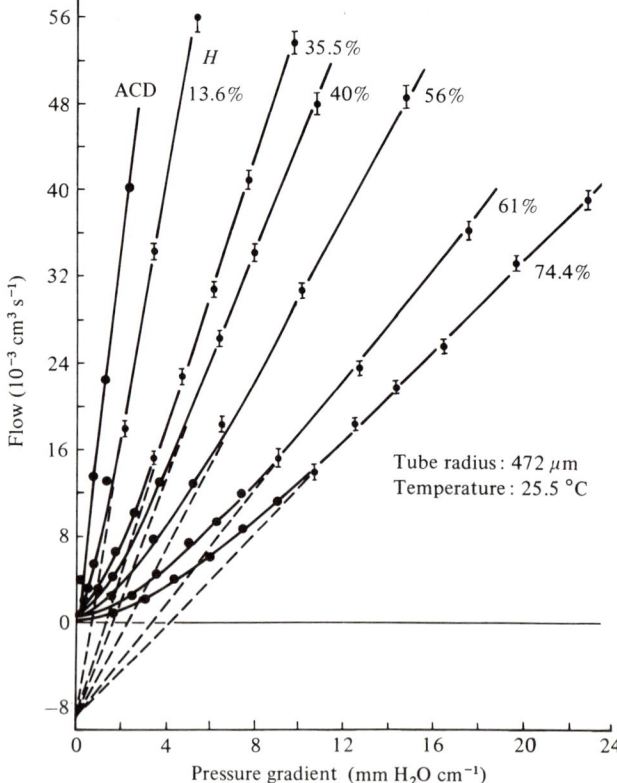

Fig. 24. Pressure–flow curves for red cell suspensions. (From Haynes & Burton, 1959.)

3.10 *Flow of red cell suspensions in small tubes*   53

has this asymptote:

$$Q = \frac{\pi R^4}{8L}\left[\frac{1}{\eta_B}\gamma^4 + \frac{1}{\eta_p}(1-\gamma^4)\right]P - \frac{\pi R^3}{3}\frac{f_B\gamma^4}{\eta_B} \qquad (3.31)$$

The second term on the right-hand side of the above equation conforms with Haynes' findings.

Doing research on the asymptotic line of the pressure–flow relationship, Inouye, Kamino, Ogawa & Uyesaka (1976) studied red cell suspension in a bull-frog's limb using perfusion. The pressure–flow curve consists of a smooth curve convex to the pressure axis, tending to a straight line at higher flow rates. The asymptotic line was found to have a negative intercept on the flow axis, which was independent of the hematocrit of the sample, and depended only on the radius of the vascular tube.

(b) Flow resistance

The flow resistance through a tube is defined by the ratio of the pressure gradient to the flow rate. There are several factors which affect the resistance of flow of red cell suspensions through small tubes. Above all, red cell aggregation and then rouleaux formation play an important role in the flow resistance at low shear rates. In fact, Palmer & Jedrzejczyk (1975) showed the significance of rouleaux formation in very slow flow through capillary channels. In order to examine the effect of cell aggregation on the flow resistance, they used 30% hematocrit human red cell suspensions in three kinds of media: (1) 0.9% NaCl, (2) 3.5% dextran 40 in 0.9 NaCl, (3) 2% dextran 200 in 0.9% NaCl. In medium (3), rouleaux formation was marked, while in (1) and (2) it was negligible; moreover, media (2) and (3) had the same viscosity. The flow resistance through capillary slits of 25 and 100 μm gap and through tubes of 400 μm and 1 mm diameter was measured for various flow rates corresponding to apparent shear rates at the wall from 20 s^{-1} to 1000 s^{-1}. In their experiments, at an apparent shear rate of 1000 s^{-1} the flow resistance was the same in media (2) and (3); at an apparent shear rate of 20 s^{-1} the flow resistance was significantly lower in medium (3) than in (1) and (2) for all capillaries. Their findings indicate that rouleaux formation reduces flow resistance in straight capillary channels with diameters from 25 to 400 μm.

Rouleaux and aggregates of red cells may of great importance in microcirculation *in vivo*. Flow energy due to pressure may be expended in breaking or forming rouleaux and aggregates at sites of branching and confluence in the microcirculation. There is no definite conclusion as to whether excess red cell aggregation impairs circulation in arterioles or venules or not.

3.11 Fahraeus effect

The flow properties of blood are strongly influenced by the hematocrit level of blood. Thus, in quantitative studies of blood flows in very small tubes and vessels, it is necessary to know how red cells are distributed in blood flows through vessels. In his classic work, Fahraeus (1929) stated that when blood flows from a large diameter tube through a capillary tube, the average hematocrit of blood in the capillary is less than that of blood in the large vessel. This phenomenon, the Fahraeus effect, is well-known.

The Fahraeus effect was quantitatively investigated by Barbee & Cokelet (1971). Let us consider their experimental studies where human blood and red cell isotonic suspensions were pumped through capillaries 29–221 μm in diameter from a large reservoir. If the hematocrit in a capillary tube and in the reservoir be denoted by H_T and H_F, respectively, the ratio of H_T to H_F is defined as the relative tube hematocrit, H_R.

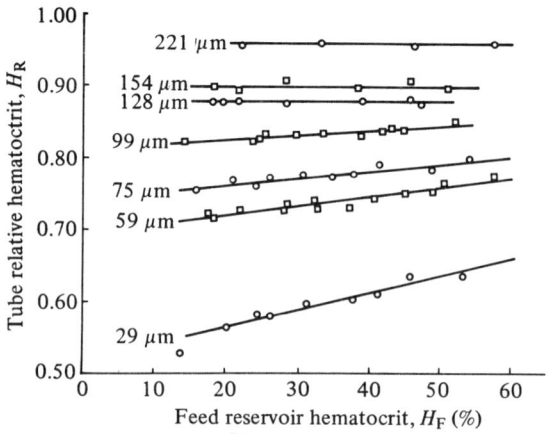

Fig. 25. H_R vs. H_F as a function of tube diameter. (From Barbee & Cokelet, 1971.)

Under steady flow conditions in the range of conditions studied, the relative tube hematocrit was found to be independent of the blood flow rate, the protein content of the continuous phase of the red cell suspension, and the stirring rate in the reservoir. Barbee & Cokelet's results are shown in Fig. 25. H_R is a linear function of H_F for a given capillary size. As the tube diameter decreases, the slope of the straight line increases, and the intercept on the ordinate decreases. The exit, mixing-cup hematocrit H_O of the blood flowing from the tube was also measured. For tubes 59 μm in diameter or larger, H_O was always equal to the feed reservoir blood hematocrit, H_F. Their results agree with those of Fahraeus ($H_F = 40\%$). It was found that the hematocrit in the capillary is a function of radial position.

The above-mentioned Fahraeus effect is interpreted as a feature of particulate flow. In a model experiment in which gelatin particles were suspended in a silicone fluid to simulate blood, Yen & Fung (1977) found that the Fahraeus effect has a point of inversion. When the diameter of the undeformed cells was equal to or greater than the tube diameter, the volume fraction of the cells in the tubes increased to a value equal to or greater than that in the reservoir.

Gaehtgens and co-workers (Gaehtgens, Albrecht & Kreutz, 1978a, Gaehtgens, Kreutz & Albrecht, 1978b) also found that the hematocrit in the discharge reservoir was markedly lower than that in the feed reservoir for red cells suspended in buffered Ringer solution passing through glass capillaries of diameter 15–95 μm. This phenomenon is probably due to the reduction in the number of red cells entering the capillary orifice. Gaehtgens *et al.* called this the '*screening effect*'. In their experiments, the cell screening increased with decreasing flow rate in the range of average shear rate $10-10^3$ s^{-1}. Moreover, in narrower capillaries of diameter 3.3–11.0 μm, the cell screening increased with decreasing diameter; a reduction of the flow rate resulted in pure plasma flow through the capillary due to the screening effect. Furthermore, it was found that the flow dependence of cell screening was intensified under the effect of dextran-induced cell aggregation.

3.12   Fahraeus–Lindqvist effect

The apparent viscosity of a non-Newtonian fluid, η'_a, is sometimes defined by means of the relation:

$$Q = \frac{\pi R^4}{8\eta'_a} \frac{\Delta p}{L} \qquad (3.32)$$

where Q is the flow rate, $\Delta p/L$ is the constant pressure gradient, and R is the inner radius of the tube through which the fluid is flowing. Note that η'_a differs from the apparent viscosity, η_a, which is defined as the ratio of the shear stress to shear rate.

It has been shown by many investigators that the apparent viscosity η'_a of blood decreases as the radius of the tube is reduced to less than about 500 μm (Fig. 26). Fahraeus & Lindqvist (1931a) were the first to study this systematically. Thus, the decrease in the apparent viscosity of blood as the tube radius is reduced is often called the *Fahraeus–Lindqvist effect*.

A similar effect has been found by rheologists in a variety of suspensions, and it is now recognized to be a general property of suspensions whose particles are the order of a micron or more in size. This reduction in the apparent viscosity with decrease in the tube diameter is usually referred to as the *sigma effect*. The term was first used by Scott Blair (1958), who named it after the Greek letter σ.

Fig. 26. Apparent viscosity of blood as a function of tube radius. △ Hess (1912); ○ Fahraeus & Lindqvist (1931b); □ Müller (1942); ● Bayliss, L. E. (unpublished). (From Bayliss, 1952.)

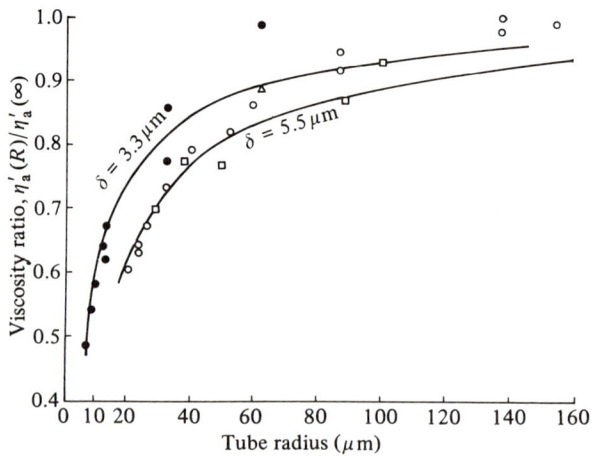

Dix & Scott Blair (1940) suggested that, if the size of suspended particles were similar to that of the tube, it would be incorrect to derive a modification of a Poiseuille's equation by integration, since the shearing layers could not be regarded as infinitely thin. Assuming that shear takes place in discontinuous layers between unsheared layers of thickness δ, the following equation is obtained:

$$\frac{\eta'_a(\infty)}{\eta'_a(R)} = \left(1 + \frac{\delta}{R}\right)^2 \quad (3.33)$$

where $\eta'_a(\infty)$ denotes the apparent viscosity for tube radius greater than 500 μm. The continuous curves in Fig. 26 are theoretical curves using this equation. No explanation is offered as to why two different groups appear to exist.

It would be too unrealistic to assume discontinuous layers in flowing suspensions in small tubes. In the case of blood, at least, a qualitative explanation for the sigma effect is possible if the existence of the plasma layer is taken into account. The plasma layer has a low coefficient of viscosity, and therefore acts as if it were a lubricant. Thus, the sigma effect becomes noticeable in small tubes where the ratio δ/R is sufficiently large. If the central core is assumed, for simplicity, to be a homogeneous Newtonian fluid of viscosity η, then we have

$$\frac{1}{\eta'_a} = \frac{1}{\eta_p} - \left(\frac{1}{\eta_p} - \frac{1}{\eta}\right)\left(1 - \frac{\delta}{R}\right)^4 \quad (3.34)$$

indicating a reduction of η'_a as R decreases. Here $\eta_p(<\eta)$ is the viscosity of the plasma layer. A similar result may be obtained from Eq. (3.28) for the central core consisting of the Casson fluid, if $(\delta/R)^2$ is much less than unity.

On the other hand, Whitmore (1959) interpreted the sigma effect in terms of the difference in hematocrit values caused by the size effect of the red cells at the entrance of the tube.

3.13 Wall surface effect – Copley–Scott Blair phenomenon

The apparent viscosity of blood measured with a capillary viscometer is influenced not only by the size of capillary tube, but also by the wall surface condition of the tube. Copley (1958, Copley & Scott Blair, 1961) reported on findings of apparent viscosity of blood, plasma and serum in contact with glass and fibrin surfaces. The apparent viscosities always showed a decrease when the blood systems were in contact with fibrin as compared with glass and other surfaces, such as silicone (Fig. 27). This wall surface effect is referred to as the Copley–Scott Blair phenomenon.

Koyama and co-workers (Koyama, Kitahara, Kanamaru & Wada, 1967, Koyama, Oki, Kanamaru & Wada, 1970, Koyama, Ooi, Wada & Kanamaru, 1971) also investigated this phenomenon; they found that fibrin lowers the apparent viscosity of blood and that the effect is more marked for blood than for plasma. This agrees with the findings of Copley, Scott Blair, Glover & Thorley (1960).

There is as yet no established theory of the Copley–Scott Blair phenomenon. Some years ago, two explanations were offered by the present writer. One is based on a slip model and the other on an electrostatic model. If it is assumed that slip occurs between the blood and the fibrin-coated walls, clearly the apparent viscosity must decrease. Let us represent the velocity and the shear stress at the tube wall by v_w and τ_w, respectively, and introduce *Oldroyd's effective slip coefficient* $\zeta = v_w/\tau_w$. Taking into account the existence of the plasma layer and assuming that the central core is a homogeneous Casson fluid, the apparent viscosity is given by the following

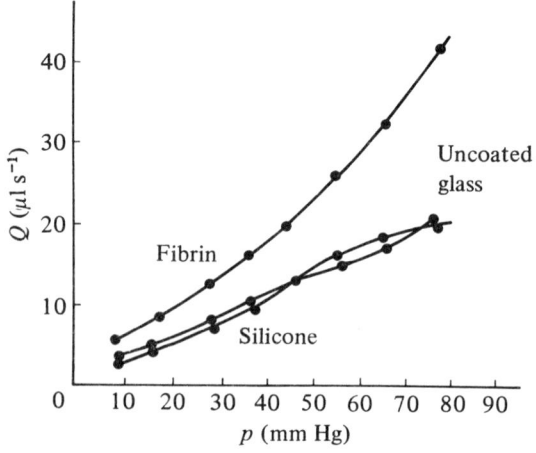

Fig. 27. Effect of fibrin coating on the pressure–flow curve. (From Copley & Scott Blair, 1961.)

3.13 Wall surface effect

equation:

$$\frac{1}{\eta'_a} = \frac{1}{\eta_c}\left(\gamma^4 - \frac{16}{7}\gamma^{7/2}\sqrt{\xi} + \frac{4}{3}\gamma^3\xi - \frac{1}{21}\xi^4\right)$$
$$+ \frac{1}{\eta_p}(1-\gamma^4) + 4\frac{\zeta}{R} \tag{3.35}$$

η'_a is obviously smaller than in the case where there is no slip ($\zeta = 0$). However, it seems difficult to find any underlying mechanism for slip between blood or plasma and the fibrin-coated wall from a molecular standpoint.

Another possibility lies in the dependence of the thickness of the plasma layer upon the wall surface condition. As is well known, red cells are covered by a membrane containing proteins such as lipoprotein, and they are negatively charged. Plasma proteins such as serum albumin, globulin, and fibrinogen are also negatively charged. It is plausible that the fibrin film on glass bears a negative charge, because the isoelectric point of fibrin s is 5.6, and fibrin i differs only slightly from fibrin s in amino acid composition. The increase of the thickness δ of the plasma layer in fibrin-coated capillaries may be caused by electrostatic repulsion between red cells and wall which pushes them towards the tube axis. Silicone, perspex, lusteroid, and paraffin exert little influence upon δ, because these substances are not polyelectrolytes. But it would be necessary to measure the increase of δ in fibrin-coated capillaries and to explain the fact quantitatively in terms of electrostatic repulsion.

Similarly, it is anticipated that the apparent viscosities will always decrease when blood is in contact with substances which are negatively charged. In fact, a reduction in the apparent viscosity of blood was observed by Ossoff & Charm (1974) when flow was through negative-charged tubing and the hematocrit was high.

A different explanation was offered by Tamamushi (1971) from the standpoint of surface chemistry. If blood or plasma flows in tubes with a fibrin-coated surface, protein molecules may be adsorbed from the plasma solution into the fibrin surface so that protein multilayers will be built up. This will result in a decrease of the protein content in plasma solution, and thus a decrease in the apparent viscosity of blood and plasma. Until the amount of adsorption is experimentally determined, it will not be known how far such a dilution effect can contribute to the decrease in viscosity of blood or plasma flowing over a fibrin-covered surface.

3.14 Disturbed flows of red cell suspensions

Red cells suspended in saline solution and plasma may affect the onset of turbulence or disturbance in flows through tubes. Stein & Sabbah (1975) studied the effects of red cells on the intensity of turbulent flow through tubes of in-vitro systems. Various red cell suspensions in a mixture of plasma and dextrose with nearly identical viscosity and density were passed through stenosed tubes in order to measure the intensity of turbulence in the flow past the stenosis. The hematocrit of red cell suspensions markedly affected the intensity of turbulence. In particular, red cell suspension at hematocrit 20–30% had over twice the turbulence intensity compared with plasma of equal viscosity and density. The addition of more cells (hematocrit 40%) resulted in a smaller difference between blood and comparable plasma. These findings strongly suggest that the presence of red cells in suspension tends to increase the turbulence in flow.

Why is turbulence increased by suspended red cells? The increase may be partly explained by the slip postulates, that non-slipping plasma is slowed down by the wall while red cells skid along the wall. Slip or non-slip flow at the wall may be partly responsible for turbulence, but the detailed mechanism remains unclear. We should note here that some materials added to liquid flows diminish the turbulence. These materials are, in general, long-chain organic compounds, such as polyethylene oxide, which reduce the flow resistance through a tube or past an obstacle. This is known as *Toms' phenomenon* (1949).

3.15 Viscosity of blood clots

(a) Thrombelastograph

The rheological behavior of blood during clotting can be examined closely with a thrombelastograph. Since this instrument was invented by Hartert (1960), it has been widely used in clinical examination of blood clotting. Basically, it consists of a rod-like cylinder hanging freely in a cylindrical container, which is oscillated sinusoidally every 3.5 s through an angle of approximately 5°

3.15 Viscosity of blood clots

around the vertical axis. The inner cylinder leaves an annular gap 1 mm wide between it and the inner wall of the container. Both container and rod are made from stainless steel. The rod is suspended on a steel wire 0.2 mm in diameter and 20 mm long. The blood which fills the annular gap transmits the motion of the container to the inner cylinder as clotting occurs. There is a small mirror attached to the rod which reflects the light of a slit lamp to record any oscillation of the rod on photographic paper moving at a constant velocity.

A typical thrombelastogram is shown in Fig. 28, where the ordinate represents the amplitude of the oscillation of the rod and the abscissa represents the time. In the thrombelastogram, the horizontal line on the left means that the blood has not yet clotted. Then there is a gradually increasing deflection of the light beam during the clotting process. Note that this instrument measures only the shear elasticity and not the viscosity of the clot.

(b) *Clotting viscoelasticity*

The blood clot exhibits strong viscoelastic properties. The apparent viscosity of blood during clotting was measured by Kaibara & Fukada (1969) using a coaxial cylinder viscometer in the shear rate range from 2 to 100 s^{-1} at room temperature. The shear rate was continuously changed to obtain the flow curve. The apparent viscosity was obtained by the equation $\eta_a = \tau/\dot{\gamma}$, where τ is the shear stress and $\dot{\gamma}$ is the shear rate. The relation between the

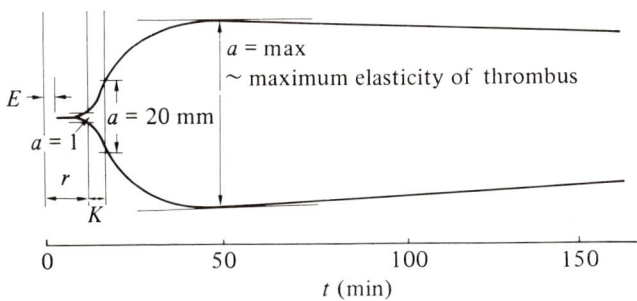

Fig. 28. Thrombelastogram. *E*: time taken to fill cell, etc; *r*: reaction time; *K*: rate of formation of fibrin clots; *a*: amplitude. (From Scott Blair, 1974.)

shear stress and shear rate during clotting accorded well with the Casson equation (Fig. 29).

The dynamic modulus and loss modulus during clotting were also measured by Kaibara & Fukada using a dynamic viscoelastic

Fig. 29. Shear-thinning behavior and Casson plot during the initial stage of clotting. (From Kaibara & Fukada, 1969.)

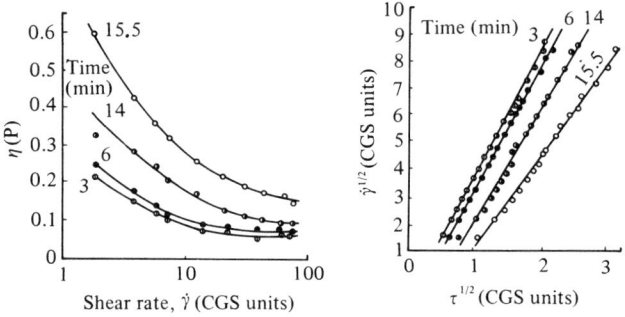

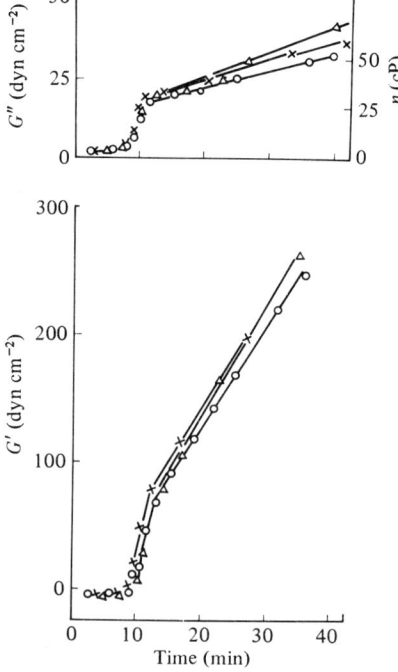

Fig. 30. Dynamic viscoelasticity of whole human blood. (From Kaibara & Fukada, 1969.)

apparatus. About 1 ml of blood was used to fill an annular gap 1 mm wide between an inner rod and a coaxial tube. The tube was made of stainless steel and had an inner diameter of 10 mm and a length of 20 mm. The rod was also made of stainless steel and had a diameter of 8 mm and the immersion depth of 20 mm. The outer cylinder was oscillated vertically by means of an electromagnetic vibrator at a frequency of 10 Hz and with a peak-to-peak amplitude of 87 μm. The inner rod was in turn oscillated vertically by the shearing force transmitted through the sample.

Figure 30 shows the dynamic modulus, G', and the loss modulus, G'', of human whole blood at the early stage of clotting for three different samples. Within a few minute of dropping a recalcifying agent on to the sample, G'' began to increase, then G'. Pharmacological alteration of coagulating whole blood may influence its rheological behavior. Overholser, Itin, Brown & Harris (1975) measured these pharmacological effects. The clot viscoelasticity was measured with a Weissenberg Rheogoniometer as a function of the concentration of the anti-coagulant sodium heparin. It was found that the elastic modulus was significantly and reproducibly lowered by heparin and that the variation between donors was minimized by adjustment of hematocrit, platelet count, and fibrinogen content to common values.

Clotting of blood is affected by the nature of the vessel surface in contact with blood. Kaibara & Fukada (1971) showed that with blood collected in a siliconized polyethylene test tube, the saturated value of G' is smaller, that of G'' is larger, and the clotting time is longer, than with blood collected in a non-siliconized glass tube.

Fukada & Kaibara (1973) later studied the dynamic shear modulus and loss modulus of solutions of fibrinogen with added thrombin, using a dynamic viscoelastic apparatus, throughout the period of gelation. They found that the dynamic modulus of fibrin gel depends upon the amplitude and frequency of oscillation applied during gelation. Mechanical agitation during gelation prevents the fibrin network from developing sufficiently.

3.16 Blood rheology at near-zero gravity

As a result of manned space flights, hemorheology at near-zero gravity has become very important. Hemorheology in astronautics was recently reviewed by Kimzey (1979). During space flight, all astronauts experience a marked reduction in the circulating red cell mass. This is probably due to the high concentration (near 100%) of oxygen inside the spacecraft. The same phenomenon was found in a chamber study in which 100% oxygen was utilized at a total pressure of 260 mm Hg.

Gravity may play an important role in blood rheology. Snyder & Seaman (1979) pointed out that gravity could affect sedimentation, buoyant convection, segregation of components through the interplay of interfacial tension, and density gradients. In biological systems, heterogeneity in size and density increases with increasing particle size. For this reason, near-zero gravity may influence biological cells markedly.

It is very difficult to measure biological cellular dispersions, especially at very low shear rate, under terrestrial conditions because of sedimentation of cells in cone–plate or coaxial cylinder viscometers. Since cell sedimentation does not occur at zero gravity, rheological studies carried out in near-zero gravity would provide new information on the effect of disparate density under low-flow conditions. This information would also pinpoint the role that gravity plays in these processes on earth. Copley (1979) considered the most important topics of hemorheology at near-zero gravity to be viscosity and elasticity of human blood in steady or oscillatory shears, viscosity and elasticity of surface layers of purified fibrinogen and other proteins, viscoelasticity and rigidity of fibrin gels. Dintenfass (1979) proposed the comparative study, under terrestrial and near-zero gravity, of the following: maximum size and morphology of human red cell aggregates, effects of various agents on the size of red cell aggregates and on the kinetics of their formation, blood viscosity under high and low shear rates.

Some peculiar phenomena will occur at near-zero gravity. In fact, Saville (1979) predicted individual features using typical examples from single phase systems. In near-zero gravity, buoyancy is diminished, but slow flows (several mm s^{-1}) are induced by surface tension. In suspensions, the sedimentation rate for an isolated particle is negligibly small, but the particle swarm moves at appreciable rates. Moreover, particles migrate across streamlines due to inertia or particle deformation, and this has cumulative effects.

3.17 Blood rheology and clinical medicine

Hematocrit is the major variable of blood viscosity. Blood viscosity is most sensitive at high hematocrits and at low shear rates, especially in the venous system and in small vessels.

In *polycythemia*, the hematocrit and the incidence of thrombosis both increase markedly. The high viscosity, the reduction in blood velocity, and local vascular disease are all responsible for vascular occlusion in polycythemia.

In anemia, on the other hand, blood viscosity decreases. The increased cardiac output in acute experimental anemia is due to the decrease in viscosity and the enhancement of myocardial contractility. One of the most important clinical problems is determining the optimal hematocrit for a patient with vascular narrowing, as in coronary artery disease.

Patients with polycythemia are prone to strokes and transient ischemic attacks. There is some evidence that increased hematocrit is closely related to cerebrovascular disease. Thomas *et al.* (1977) investigated cerebral blood flow and viscosity in patients without polycythemia but with hematocrit values around the generally accepted upper limit of normality. The found cerebral blood flow in patients with hematocrits of 47–53% was significantly lower than in patients with hematocrits of 36–46%. After reducing the hematocrit in the higher group by venesection, cerebral blood flow increased by approximately 50%. This improvement in flow was largely due to a reduction in viscosity. Thus they concluded that a hematocrit around the generally accepted upper limit of normality may be an important cause of occlusive cerebrovascular disease.

Many people are continuously exposed to the high level of carbon monoxide in tobacco smoke. The inhaled carbon monoxide has a marked affinity for hemoglobin, and is readily measurable as blood carboxyhemoglobin. This preferential binding of carbon monoxide to hemoglobin replaces oxygen and produces an increased affinity between the remaining oxygen and hemoglobin molecules. Thus, excessive and sustained exposure to carbon monoxide from *smoking* produces hypoxemia, which can, in turn, cause polycythemia.

Considerable evidence has accumulated to link smoking and polycythemia. Smith & Landaw (1978) concluded that exposure to carbon monoxide from tobacco smoke is a frequent cause of an elevated red cell volume or a reduced plasma volume (or both). Measurement of carboxyhemoglobin should be a routine part of the evaluation of all polycythemic patients.

Significant and critical changes in blood flow may result from alterations in plasma proteins, especially fibrinogen. These alterations are responsible for red cell aggregation, especially at low shear. Abnormal serum proteins may occasionally be of marked importance in viscosity. A hyperviscosity syndrome has been described in *macroglobulinemia* and in *multiple myeloma*.

Supplement to Sect. 3.13 (added in proof)

Consider a Newtonian liquid containing ions flowing steadily through a tube of radius R and length L under a constant pressure difference Δp. If the existence of an *electric double layer* at the solid–liquid interface is taken into consideration, it may be shown that the flow rate Q is given by

$$Q = \frac{\pi R^4}{8\eta} \frac{\Delta p}{L}(1 + \alpha) \qquad \alpha = \frac{\varepsilon}{2\pi} \frac{\sigma \zeta}{Kn} \frac{1}{R}$$

where η, ε and K are the viscosity, the dieletric constant and the specific conductance, respectively, of the liquid; σ is the surface charge density at the interface and ζ is the *zeta potential*. The apparent viscosity η_a is then given by $\eta_a = \eta/(1 + \alpha)$ so that η_a decreases with increase in $\sigma\zeta$.

The above generalized relationship may be applied to a reasonable explanation of the Copley–Scott Blair phenomenon. Note that the explanation is valid not only for blood, but also for plasma and serum.

4

Red cell deformability

4.1 Red cell deformability

The red blood cell, a biconcave disc when at rest, readily changes in shape when subjected to mechanical influences. The deformations are very transient, and the red cell recovers its original shape easily after removal of external forces. Observations of the capillary bed have revealed various shapes of red cells: for example, parachute- or bullet-like.

Red cell deformability is very important in blood circulation. It allows the passage of red cells through capillaries with diameters smaller than that of the biconcave disc. Note that the severest restriction that exists, particularly in the passage through the spleen, is approximately 3 μm mean diameter. Thus, the red cell deformability plays an important role in the blood circulation in microvessels. In addition, it is due to the high deformability of red cells that blood can circulate easily even in small vessels, in spite of the large hematocrit values of 40–45%.

The shear-thinning behavior of blood is thought to result from the alignment of the major axis of the elongated cell in the direction of flow. In fact, hardening of red cells by treatment with glutaraldehyde eliminates the shear-thinning behavior. This can be explained by the larger hydrodynamic effective volume of the hardened cell rotating in the shear flow (Fig. 31).

Red cell deformability plays an important role in the blood circulation not only in microvessels, but also in blood vessels whose lumen is markedly diminished by atherosclerosis or thrombosis. A decrease in red cell deformability causes an increase in the viscosity of blood, and consequently a decrease in the flow rate. This in turn causes a diminution of the shear rate and the oxygen supply to the tissues, resulting in an increase in the blood viscosity; thus, a vicious circle arises.

One of the most striking findings about red cell deformability is the phenomenon of *tank tread motion* of the red cell membrane discovered by Fischer & Schmid-Schönbein (1978). Single cells suspended in viscous solutions, for example, dextran under shear, are deformed into flat ellipsoids. Their elongation approaches a maximum with increasing shear stress; the membrane shows tank tread motion, the frequency of which increases linearly with the shear rate (Fig. 32).

4.2 Red cell morphology

(a) Shape

The shape of a red blood cell is generally a biconcave disc, but in a normal population of red cells there is a considerable variation in both size and shape. The mean dimensions of normal red cells are: diameter = 8.1 μm, greatest thickness = 2.7 μm,

Fig. 31. Streamlines around a suspended particle. (*a*) rigid sphere, (*b*) hardened red cell, (*c*) normal red cell at high shear. (From Chien, 1975.)

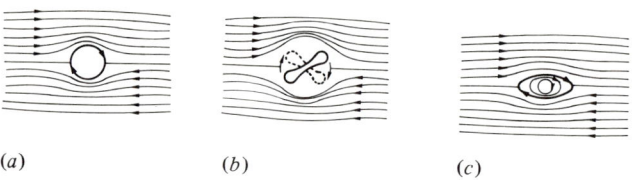

(*a*)   (*b*)   (*c*)

Fig. 32. Tank treading frequency vs. shear rate. (From Fischer & Schmid-Schönbein, 1978.)

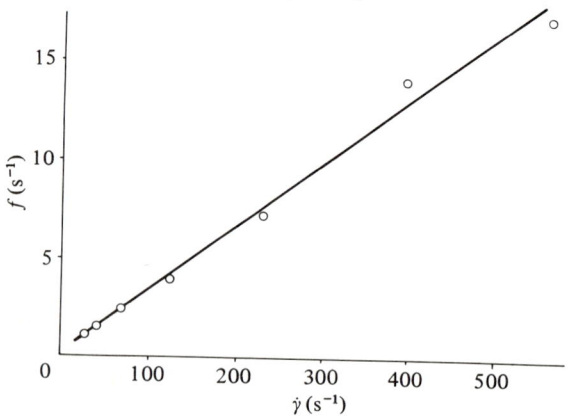

4.2 Red cell morphology

least thickness = 1.0 μm, area = 138 μm², and volume = 95 μm³ (Burton, 1972).

Special attention has been paid to the particular shape of red cells by many investigators, but the reason for the shape is not yet clear. It was postulated that the dimples are attracted by filamentous material (probably protein fibers) inside the red cell; but this cannot be the reason, because a ghost cell returns to its original shape. Since a red cell can regain its original shape after hemolysis, it can be assumed that hemoglobin does not contribute to the shape of the red cell. It has often been pointed out that a shape which allows diffusion to the innermost parts in the shortest time is advantageous. Although the biconcave disc shape provides for faster diffusion than a sphere, this still does not explain the shape, because a flatter disc of larger diameter would permit even faster diffusion. It is well-known that a red cell is negatively charged. It was postulated that the biconcave disc shape is an equipotential surface; but it is difficult to regard the red cell as an electric conductor.

Another view is that the biconcave shape represents the shape in which the total energy of bending of the membrane is minimum for a given value of the volume and surface area of a red cell. Let us consider various shapes of cells under the conditions that both volume and surface area are constant. The cells are covered by elastic membranes so that an elastic energy can be attributed to each shape of the cell. Canham (1970) studied what is called Cassini's oval, i.e. a closed surface which is generated by rotating the curve

$$y = B[(C^4 + 4A^2x^2)^{1/2} - A^2 - x^2]^{1/2} \quad (4.1)$$

around the y-axis, where A, B, C are parameters. A group of closed surfaces are obtained subject to the conditions of appropriate constant volume and surface area, each surface having the strain energy of bending

$$U = \frac{Eh^3}{24(1-\sigma^2)} \int \left(\frac{1}{R_1^2} + \frac{1}{R_2^2} \right) dS \quad (4.2)$$

where h is the thickness of the membrane, E is Young's modulus, σ is Poisson's ratio, R_1 and R_2 are the principal radii of curvature, and the integration is made over the total surface area. Since U contains the parameter B, a definite strain energy and shape are attributed to each value of B (Fig. 33). Canham minimized the surface integral U, and the solution turned out to look very much like the biconcave disc. Thus, he concluded that the cell is biconcave to minimize the strain energy of bending of the cell membrane.

Equation (4.2) is based on the assumption that the unstrained state is a flat plate, i.e. $U = 0$ when $R_1 = R_2 = \infty$. If the equilibrium shape of a red cell is unstrained, Canham's theory is not valid (Fung, 1977); stretching energy is not taken into account. Fung showed that in deforming a thin plate of diameter 8 μm and wall thickness 100 Å into a biconcave shell like a red cell, the strain energy for stretching is much larger than that for bending.

Generally speaking, a thin solid body allows a large deformation without increase of the surface area, whereas a spherical solid body can only be deformed slightly, because a sphere has a minimum surface area under a given volume. Thus, the surface area to volume ratio S/V is usually considered as a factor affecting the deformability of red cells. Note that this ratio is not a dimensionless parameter, but has the dimension $[L]^{-1}$, indicating that the ratio S/V decreases as the size of the red cell increases.

It is convenient to introduce the *sphericity index* (s.i.)

$$\text{s.i.} = 4.84 \, V^{2/3}/S \tag{4.3}$$

which is dimensionless and does not depend on size. In the above,

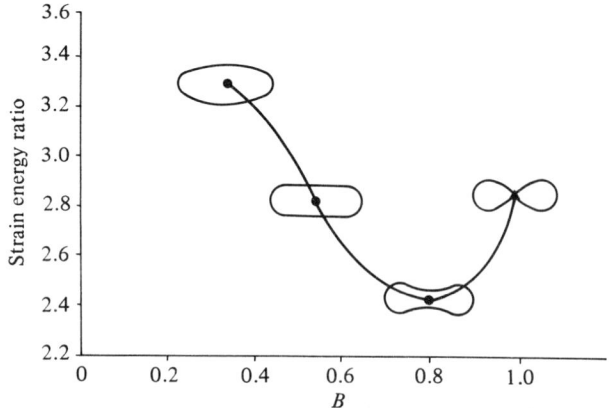

Fig. 33. Strain energy vs. parameter B of Cassini's oval. (From Canham, 1970.)

4.2 Red cell morphology

the factor 4.84 is introduced so that the index is unity for a sphere. The sphericity index of all other shapes is less than unity.

(b) *Membrane structure*

Like all other cells, the red blood cell is surrounded by a membrane. The membrane accounts for only some 3% of the human red cell. Its thickness appears to be between 60 and 200 Å. Examination of the membrane of red cell ghosts with a polarization microscope indicates a surface ultrastructure. Such studies produced the classic model of Danielli and Davson (1935), consisting of a lipid bilayer covered by a layer of protein molecules.

Singer & Nicolson (1972) proposed the *'fluid mosaic model'* of biomembranes (Fig. 34). They suggested that the proteins are predominantly globular, with their hydrophilic ends protruding from the membrane and their hydrophobic ends embedded in the lipid bilayer. Some of the proteins are simply embedded on one side or the other, while others pass entirely through the bilayer.

It has been shown that a net of fibrous protein molecules, *spectrin*, is loosely spread over the whole inner surface of the red cell membrane (Fig. 35). Thus, the spectrin network could provide the high shear resistance which the membrane exhibits at large

Fig. 34. A diagram of the fluid mosaic model (From Singer, 1975.)

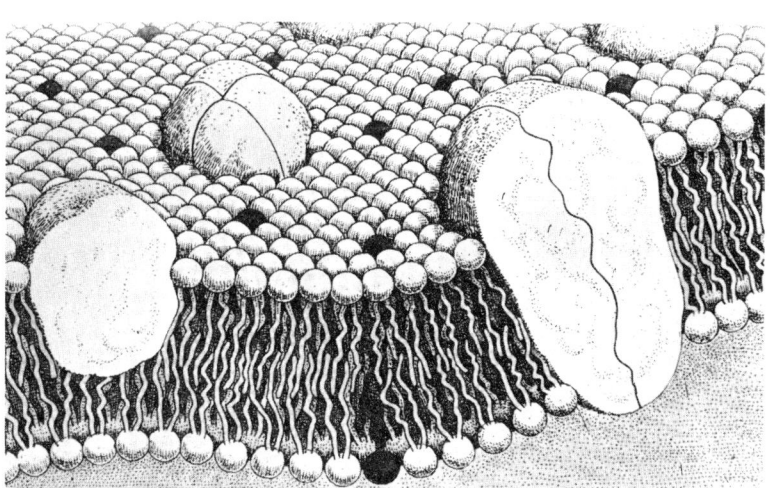

deformations. There are several reasons why the red cell would be expected to need special reinforcement of this sort. First, the red cell floats free without mechanical support from neighboring cells. Second, it is subject to a mechanical deformation as it is forced through finer capillaries. Third, the biconcave shape speeds the process of oxygen intake and release. Thus, a spectrin scaffolding seems to help the red cell retain, or rapidly regain, the characteristic shape in the face of the special stresses to which it is subjected.

The red blood cell has been particularly useful for the study of membrane properties. Recent work on the localization of membrane components in the red blood cell has indicated that the membrane appears to consist of an asymmetric lipid bilayer and an asymmetric distribution of membrane protein. The major portion of the membrane protein appears to be on the cytoplasmic face, while a smaller part of the protein goes through the lipid layer or is present solely on the external face. A variation of the older model originally proposed by Danielli & Davson, the 'fluid mosaic model' of Singer & Nicolson (1972), was recently put forward largely on the basis of experiments on the fluidity of membrane components. However, Blank & Britten (1975) concluded that the red cell membrane was probably thicker and less fluid, at least in parts, than was suggested

Fig. 35. A diagram of the undersurface of a red cell membrane A: spectrin network; B, C: globular protein molecules. (From Bull, 1978.)

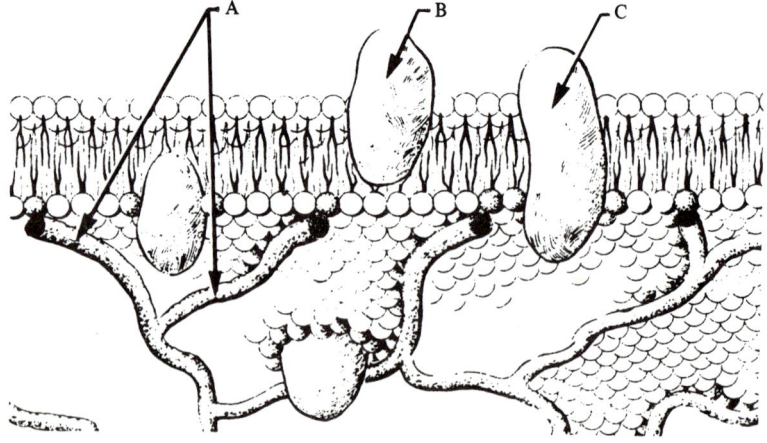

in the fluid mosaic model. The external lipid bilayer of the membrane, which can regulate the passive permeability of the cell, is probably relatively fluid. But in addition there is probably a more rigid protein layer of about the same thickness, which, though quite permeable, gives the cell membrane its structural integrity.

4.3 Measuring techniques

Various methods for measuring red cell deformability have been developed. Chien (1978a) classified them into three major categories: (1) methods for investigating cells in free suspension; (2) methods for investigating cells partially attached (flow channel methods); and (3) methods for investigating cells passing through narrow channels. Each category includes several techniques. The spin label technique is also added. Each technique has its own advantages and disadvantages, and a combination of these techniques is needed for further study of red cell deformability.

(1a) Viscometry

Red cell deformability can be tested indirectly by viscometric measurements of cell suspensions. The rotational viscometer, i.e. a coaxial cylinder viscometer or a cone–plate viscometer, is preferable, because measurements with this instrument can be

Fig. 36. Red cell deformability and apparent viscosity of red cell suspensions. (From Chien, 1978a.)

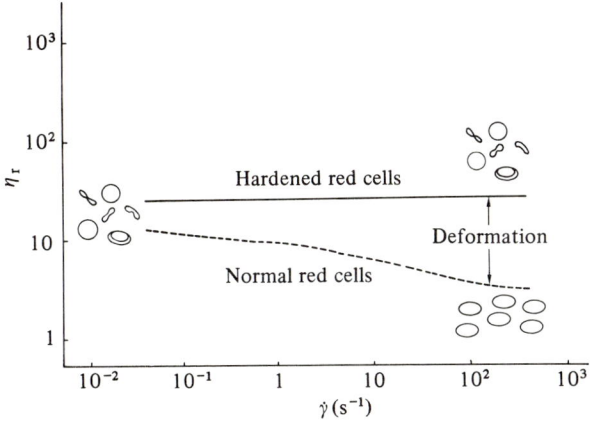

made not only at various shear rates, but also under oscillatory conditions.

Chien (1978a) showed the effect of red cell deformability on the viscosity of a suspension of red cells. The viscosity of a suspension of normal red cells in Ringer–albumin solution at controlled cell concentration (for example, 45%) decreases as the shear rate increases, whereas the viscosity of a suspension of hardened red cells treated with glutaraldehyde at the same concentration shows no change with the shear rate (Fig. 36). The lowering of the viscosity of normal red cells at high shear rates is attributed to the alignment of red cells due to the deformation.

(1*b*) *Counter-rotating rheoscope*

In order to study the deformability of red cells quantitatively, microscopic observation of the behavior of red cells subject to quantifiable shear stress is desirable. Schmid-Schönbein used a counter-rotating rheoscope for this purpose (Fig. 37). The principal

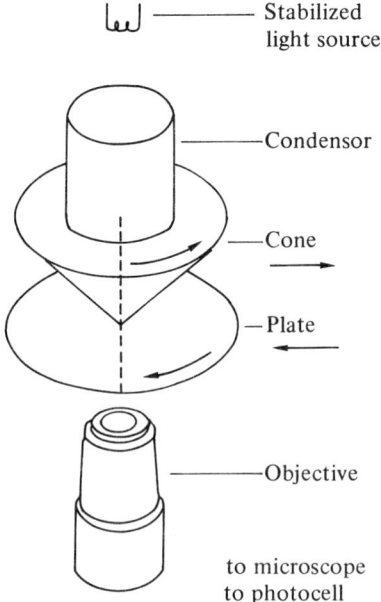

Fig. 37. Counter-rotating rheoscope. (From Schmid-Schönbein *et al.* 1973.)

parts are a transparent glass plate mounted on a rotating support, and a flat transparent Plexiglas cone rotating around the cone axis in the opposite direction to the plate, and at the same angular velocity. In the middle, between the plate and the cone, red cells remain stationary to the observer, while they are subjected to quantifiable shear stress. In order to increase the shear stress, high molecular weight dextran is added. At shear stresses above 3 dyn cm^{-2}, red cells are not biconcave, but are elongated like an ellipsoid and oriented with their major axes parallel to the flow. Further studies led to the conclusion that the red cell membrane is in perpetual tank tread motion around the fluid cell content during such deformation. Evidence of such membrane rotation is now available (Fig. 31).

(1c) *Diffractometric method* (*Ektacytometer*)

Bessis & Mohandas (1975) describe a technique to measure the deformability of red cells, in which the cell suspension is subjected to well-defined shear stresses in a concentric cylinder viscometer, and the elongation of the cell is measured using diffractometry. The advantage of this technique is that cellular deformability of a population of cells can be measured rapidly using extremely small quantities of blood (50 μl of whole blood).

The concentric cylinder viscometer consists of a fixed Plexiglas inner cylinder and a rotating outer cylinder (Fig. 38). The diameter of the inner cylinder is 50 mm and the gap between the cylinders is

Fig. 38. Ektacytometer. (From Bessis & Mohandas, 1975.)

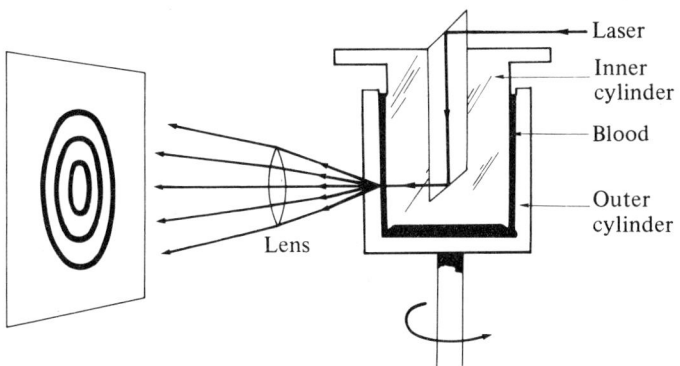

0.5 mm. The rate of revolution of the outer cylinder can be varied from 0 to 100 revolutions per minute (RPM). The shear stress is then given by

$$\tau = \frac{2\pi \eta N R}{60 h} \quad (\text{dyn cm}^{-2}) \tag{4.4}$$

where R is the radius of the inner cylinder, h is the gap between the cylinders, and N is the RPM of the outer cylinder. η is the suspending medium viscosity, which is varied by changing the amount of dextran 40 (average molecular weight 40 000) in the solutions in order to obtain large shear stresses.

To obtain the diffraction patterns, a helium–neon laser source is used and, with the aid of two prisms, the beam is made to traverse the gap between the two cylinders. It is observed that the diffraction pattern of red cells under conditions of no stress is circular. When the cells are deformed by the fluid shear stresses, the diffraction patterns become elliptical (Fig. 39). The cellular length d can be obtained from

$$d = \frac{a_0}{a} d_0 \tag{4.5}$$

where d_0 is the diameter of the cells under conditions of no stress, a_0 is the diameter of the first diffraction ring at no stress, and a is the minor axis dimension of the elliptical pattern.

Allard, Mohandas & Bessis (1978) showed that the diffraction patterns at 125 dyn cm^{-2} of blood samples obtained by mixing

Fig. 39. Diffraction patterns of normal human red cells at various shear rates. (From Bessis & Mohandas, 1975.)

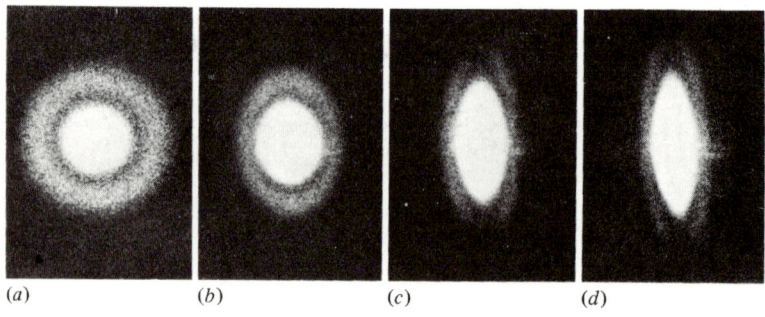

(a)   (b)   (c)   (d)

normally deforming cells with various proportions of undeformable glutaraldehyde-fixed cells produce a composite pattern in which an elliptic pattern is superimposed upon a circular pattern. The intensity of the pattern in the elliptical and circular portions is directly proportional to the percentage of these two populations.

(1d) *Centrifugal packing*

The packing of red cells when subjected to centrifugal force is closely related to their deformability. Chien *et al.* (1968) showed that normal red cells can be packed to nearly 100% after 5 min of centrifugation at 15000g, while red cells hardened with acetaldehyde or glutaraldehyde can be packed to only 60%.

(2a) *Floor attachment method*

This technique was developed by Hochmuth, Mohandas & Blackshear (1973) to study the stress–strain relationship of red cells. A rectangular flow channel is constructed, and fluid flows between two parallel surfaces designed to be 100 μm apart. A dilute red cell suspension is introduced into the channel. After allowing 15 min for the red cells to settle to the floor of the channel, the cell-free suspending medium is pumped through the channel at a constant rate. A red cell which appears to adhere to the floor at a single point is referred to as having a 'point attachment', while a cell which is attached to the floor at two or more points is referred to as having a 'line attachment'. The degree of cell elongation at different flow rates is determined by microphotography, and the shear stress acting on the upper surface of the cell can be calculated approximately by

$$\tau = \frac{h}{2d}\Delta p \qquad (4.6)$$

where Δp is the pressure drop, d is the distance between the inlet and outlet, and h is the channel height. Figure 40 shows the elongation of two red cells as a function of the shear stress at the wall for the two different types of attachment.

The flow channel method was originally used to measure the elastic properties of cells. But it can also be used to measure plastic deformation, and viscoelastic behavior of the cell membrane.

(2b) Fiber-arrest method

Bull, Brailsford & Korpman (1978) developed this technique to study cell deformability. A cell, arrested on a fibrin strand, is elongated by rapidly moving fluid. Where the membrane trap crosses the fine fiber, it narrows as the fluid velocity increases, because the total area of the cell membrane remains constant. The relationship of trap width to deforming force is used as a measure of membrane deformability (Fig. 41). Note that it is difficult to determine quantitatively the force produced by the moving fluid.

(3a) Micropipette method

Aspiration with a micropipette is a technique that has been widely used to measure the deformability of cells. The more easily the cell is aspirated, the more deformable it is. There are three

Fig. 40. Elongation of red cells in floor attachment method. (a) point attachment, (b) line attachment. (From Hochmuth et al., 1973.)

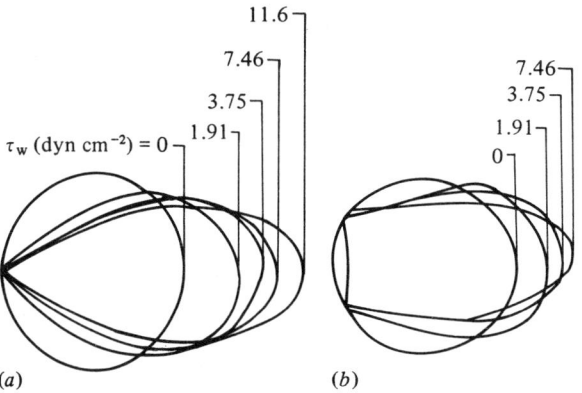

Fig. 41. Elongation of red cell in fiber-arrest method. (From Bull et al., 1978.)

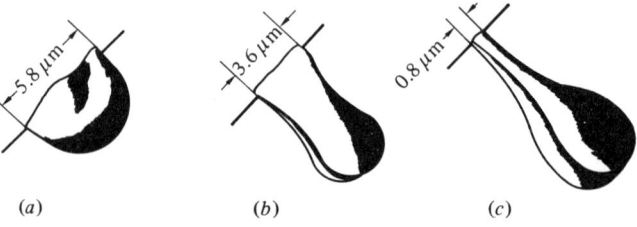

methods (Fig. 42). The first is to measure the negative pressure in millimeters of water required to induce a standard 1 μm penetration of the cell's surface into a 1.5 μm diameter glass pipette. The second is to measure the distance of penetration in μm of a portion of the cell into the same 1.5 μm pipette at a fixed pressure difference of 3 mm of water. The third, which assesses the deformability of the whole cell, measures the negative pressure needed to induce complete penetration into a 2.8 to 3.0 μm diameter pipette.

The micropipette technique, unlike the other techniques, can measure the deformability of individual cells. By measuring the time course of deformation or recovery of a cell in response to sudden pressure changes via a micropipette, one can obtain the time constant, i.e. the retardation time, by using a simple Kelvin model.

It is generally accepted that the micropipette technique measures the membrane elasticity of a cell, but it is not clear whether this is extensional elasticity or bending elasticity. The deformation of a cell membrane in the micropipette test is rather complicated, and there is probably a significant bending resistance near the micropipette tip. The micropipette technique probably measures the composite effect of both bending and extensional elasticity.

(3b) *Filtration method*

Red cell deformability can be studied by determining the percentage of cells passing through a filter at a given pressure gradient. There are three general types of filters employed in these studies.

Fig. 42. Aspiration of a red cell in micropipette method. (From Leblond, 1973.)

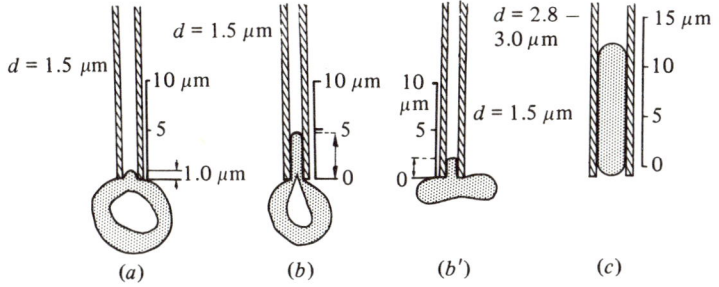

(i) Paper-fiber filters

These have long multibranching channels with dimensions approximately equal to the red cell diameter, and a thickness many times greater than the cell diameter.

(ii) Millipore filters

These consist of an inert matrix penetrated by tubular channels having greater uniformity of diameter and virtually no branching compared with paper filters.

(iii) Polycarbonate sieves

These consist of polycarbonate membranes of less than 15 μm thickness through which right cylindrical channels of very uniform dimensions have been produced by X-irradiation.

Sieves with 3 μm pore diameter are most useful, since this is about the critical size for passage of normal human red cells. Sieves with 5 μm pore diameter are more suitable for red cells with markedly reduced deformability. The pore diameter of each sieve should be checked by microscopic measurements.

Note that the passage of red cells through filters differs from that through microvessels because of the nature of artificial materials.

Electron spin resonance can be used to study molecular motion of cell membranes, which is closely related to cell deformability. This method is suitable for molecules with unpaired electrons. For a single electron, the spin is either parallel or antiparallel to the magnetic field. The energy difference between these two is: $\Delta E = g\mu H$, where g is the Landé factor, μ is the spin magnetic moment of one electron, and H is the magnetic field. If a photon of exactly this energy ΔE is applied, it will be absorbed, flipping an electron spin from antiparallel to parallel; i.e. there is a resonance at a frequency:

$$v = g\mu H/h \qquad (4.7)$$

where h is Planck's constant. It is possible to measure the magnetic field H that makes a fixed frequency v the resonant one. It is also possible to measure the breadth of the absorption peaks, which indicates the strength of the interactions with neighboring groups of atoms; the breadth gives us information about the molecular motion of the system; the sharper the peak is, the nearer the system is to the liquid state.

The *spin label technique* has been widely used to investigate molecular phenomena in biological membranes. The motion parameter of the incorporated spin label is frequently used as a measure of the membrane lipid phase, and is consequently employed as an index of membrane fluidity.

Shiga *et al.* (1979b) demonstrated the decreased membrane fluidity of aged, human red cells by monitoring the electron spin resonance spectra of fatty acid spin labels in the membrane. The decrease of ATP in the aged cells and their decreased deformability, were also shown. The alteration of the protein–lipid organization, and/or the effects of the diminished ATP content, are thought to cause the decreased membrane fluidity of aged red cells *in vivo*.

4.4 Factors affecting red cell deformability

Red cell deformability is influenced by the following factors:

(a) *Membrane elasticity*

It is obvious that the smaller the membrane elasticity, the more the red cell is deformable. But when we speak of elastic modulus, we must distinguish between extensional modulus, shear modulus (rigidity), and bending modulus; the bending modulus is not purely a material constant, but the product of Young's modulus and the moment of inertia of a cross-section around a neutral line.

Kumar (1976) showed from a qualitative analysis that it was better to consider blood as a heterogeneous medium in order that the combined behavior of red cells and plasma should correspond to the rheological behavior of blood. The existence of an elastic membrane over the deformable red cell means that when flowing with the plasma the membrane could absorb energy intended for the flow process. He further suggested that during the momentum transport computation it is necessary to recognize both a pure alignment process and an alignment with deformation process for the red cell. He contended that energy is supplied for the latter process, and that the energy supplied could be released by the membranes of red cells. This energy, when released, is responsible for the random movement, the collisions, the orientation and the disaggregation of red blood cells. Once that energy is accounted for, the above-mentioned processes do not need any energy.

(b) Membrane viscoelasticity

Generally speaking, red cell membranes exhibit viscoelasticity rather than elasticity. The viscous component may be consistent with the fluid mosaic model proposed for biological membranes by Singer & Nicolson (1972).

(c) Internal viscosity and osmotic pressure

In red cells, both membranes and cell contents undergo deformation. The cell content is a solution containing hemoglobin, and its viscosity is referred to as '*internal viscosity*'. Red cell deformability decreases as the internal viscosity increases.

Suspending red cells in a hypotonic medium causes cell swelling, and the internal viscosity decreases. On the other hand, suspending them in a hypertonic medium causes cell shrinkage, and the internal viscosity increases. Thus, the change of internal viscosity is accompanied by the deformation of cell membranes. It seems difficult to determine separately the internal viscosity, and membrane elasticity.

(d) ATP content

Nakao, M. Nakao, T. & Yamazoe (1960) demonstrated that ATP is essential to maintain the biconcave disc shape of normal red blood cells. Weed, LaCelle & Merrill (1969), using the micropipette technique, found that ATP and Ca^{2+} played an important role in the cell shape and deformability. In a review article, LaCelle (1971) also describes the important direct effect of ATP in maintaining the marked deformability as well as the advantageous biconcave disc shape of the red cell.

Meiselman & Baker (1977) studied the rheological behavior of ATP-depleted human red cells and the influence of red blood cell morphology on the flow behavior of these cell suspensions. ATP depletion via 24h incubation at 37°C caused: (i) red blood cell crenation (discocyte-echinocyte); (ii) increased low shear rate viscosity; (iii) enhanced non-Newtonian flow behavior.

Disagreeing with the above results, Feo & Mohandas (1978) concluded from their experiments that the shape of the red cell was not directly dependent on the presence of intracellular ATP molecules, and that the deformability appeared to be independent of the intracellular ATP level and only dependent on the shape of the cells.

(e) Cholesterol content

Shiga et al. (1979a) studied the influence of the membrane cholesterol on the rheological and functional properties of the human red cells. As the cholesterol–phospholipid molar ratio is artificially increased, (i) the viscosity of the red cell suspension slightly increases; (ii) the deformability, expressed by the 'easiness' to enter into a small orifice, decreases; (iii) the rate of the oxygen egress from the red cells is retarded. These changes may be primarily due to the condensing effect of cholesterol in the lipid portion of the cell membrane, because the other biochemical and morphological factors among the samples were similar.

(f) Oxygen tension

LaCelle (1971) observed that whereas the red cell membrane retains its extremely deformable character down to P_{O_2} values of 30 mm Hg, any further decrease results in a marked stiffness of the red cell. The rigidity associated with lowered oxygen tension was interpreted to be a consequence of hemoglobin binding of ATP with resultant diminution of the ATP concentration at the inner membrane surface and concomitant calcium-induced stiffening.

Chien (1978b) studied the rheological behavior of Hb SS blood, cell suspensions and cell content in the oxygenated state and following controlled deoxygenation. Oxygenated Hb SS blood had higher viscosity than Hb AA blood at the same hematocrit, and this is attributable to (i) an elevated plasma viscosity; (ii) a higher intracellular viscosity due to elevated mean corpuscular hemoglobin concentration; (iii) cell membrane rigidity. The viscosity of suspensions of Hb SS cells began to rise with minor degrees of O_2 desaturation. Microsieving through 5 μm pores is more sensitive than viscometry in detecting the reduced deformability of slightly deoxygenated Hb SS cells. The results suggest that low flow states

Red cell deformability 84

in sickle cell disease may lead to a vicious circle not only by decreasing the tissue O_2 tension, but also by reducing the shear stress needed for cell deformation.

4.5 Significance of deformability in blood flow
(a) Occlusive arterial disease

Ehrly (1975) proposed a new therapeutic approach in occlusive arterial disease based on a hemorheological principle. In spite of occlusion or stenosis, the flow rate of blood can be increased by improving the blood's flow properties in several ways. One way is to reduce red cell aggregation. Another way is to improve the deformability of red cells.

In the microcirculation of an exercising muscle, a local hyperosmolarity was found. Blood hyperosmolarity causes shrinkage of the red cell membrane (crenated cells) and thereby decreases the

Fig. 43. Effect of pentoxifyllin on the filterability of hyperosmolar blood. (*a*) structural formula of pentoxifyllin, (*b*) filterability of blood. (From Ehrly, 1975.)

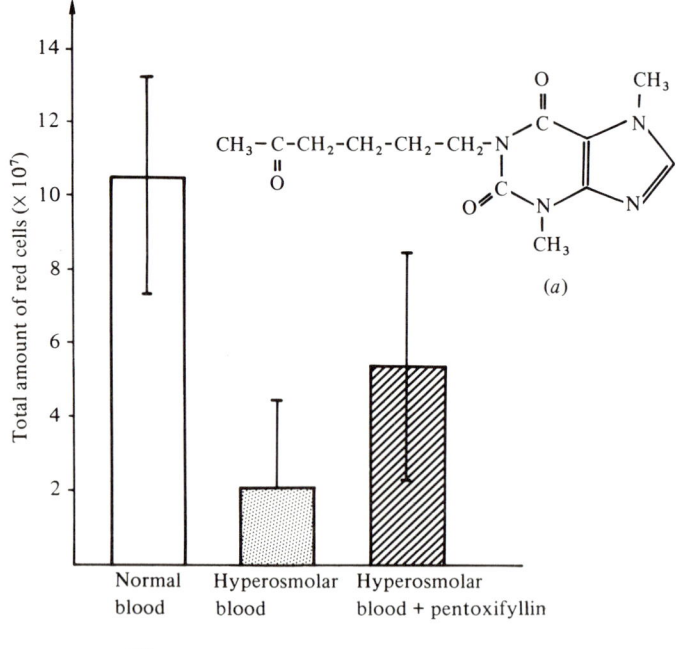

deformability of red cells. The addition of pentoxifyllin 3, 7-dimethyl-1-(5-oxohexyl)-xanthine, a vasoactive substance, to blood *in vitro* was found to increase the deformability of red cells in hyperosmolar blood samples by increasing their cellular ATP content. Thus, the reduced flow rate of hyperosmolar blood through standardized 8 μm Millipore filter could be more than doubled by the addition of pentoxifyllin (Fig. 43).

It should be noted that normal blood flow is not improved by pentoxifyllin. More needs to be known about the mechanism which improves the red cell deformability.

It was later shown that isoxsuprine, an adrenalin derivative with a vasodilator action, gave rise to a statistically significant decrease in blood viscosity *in vivo* as well as *in vitro*. The decrease of viscosity was greater at lower than at higher shear rates. Plasma viscosity and serum viscosity also fell, but to a lesser degree. There was no effect on the hematocrit. The decrease in blood viscosity is probably due to a decrease in the tendency to aggregate and an increase in the deformability of red cells.

(b) Turbulent blood flow

Sabbah & Stein (1976) studied *in vitro* the effect of red cell deformability upon turbulent blood flow. Fresh blood and blood composed of hardened cells from four healthy volunteers was passed through a precision orifice at rates sufficient to produce turbulence. Flow was steady, with a duration of 0.5–2.5 s. The random fluctuations of velocity indicative of turbulent flow were measured with a hot-film probe. At all Reynolds numbers studied, suspensions of normally deformable cells consistently showed lower turbulence than suspensions of cells made non-deformable by glutaraldehyde. The viscoelastic properties of the membranes of normal red cells appeared to cause the red cells to act as an energy sink by absorbing some of the kinetic energy generated by turbulent flow. The results of this study may be of clinical significance in view of the possible pathophysiological effects of turbulent blood flow.

4.6 Red cell deformability and clinical medicine

Red cell deformability is of considerable significance in

clinical medicine. It is critical in microvessels and at high hematocrits.

In *sickle-cell disease*, an abnormally structured hemoglobin causes the red cell membrane to conform to its sickle-like shape. Resistance to capillary flow in the sickle-cell disorders is related to decreased deformability of red cells. The deformability of sickle cells lies between that of hardened cells and normal cells. Increased blood viscosity leads to initiation of the vicious circle with subsequent stasis, hypoxia, sickle transformation and vaso-occlusion. In sickle-cell disease, thrombosis often occurs, particularly in the kidney.

The shape of red cells is closely related to the deformability, which, in turn, affects the blood viscosity. In diseases such as *elliptocytosis* and *spherocytosis*, the cells tend to become more compact and spherical. In such diseases the deformability may be decreased and viscosity may be raised nearer to Newtonian levels.

In diseases such as those associated with sickle-cell anemia, severe burns, hemorrhage, noradrenalin infusion, high butterfat intake and exposure to hypertonic saline, the cell surface becomes crenated, and the viscosity may be increased, possibly due to the increase in effective volume of the cells.

5

Rheology of microcirculation

5.1 Significance of rheology in microcirculation

In microcirculation, i.e. circulation of blood in microvessels, Reynolds numbers are very small. In fact, they are 0.02, 0.002 and 0.007, respectively, for the arteriole, capillary and venule of the dog. This indicates that in microcirculation the effect of inertia is negligible compared with that of blood viscosity. The pulsatile nature in the pressure and flow almost disappears in microcirculation; the flow may be regarded approximately as a steady one. (This corresponds to the fact that the Womersley parameter α (see Chapter 7) is also very small in microcirculation.)

Because of the effect of blood viscosity, the mechanical energy loss, i.e. the pressure drop, in microcirculation is remarkable. Consequently, blood flows very slowly. For instance, the mean velocities in the arteriole, capillary and venule of the dog are 0.3, 0.07 and 0.07 cm s^{-1}, respectively. Under such circumstances, the non-Newtonian behavior of blood plays a more significant role than in large blood vessels.

One of the characteristics of microcirculation is that blood cannot be regarded as a homogeneous continuous fluid. In microvessels, such as arterioles and venules, the existence of the plasma layer must be taken into account. In capillaries, whose diameters approach the size of the red blood cells, the particulate nature of blood becomes important.

From the physiological point of view, the most important function of circulation is to supply nutrients to every living cell of the organism and also to remove various waste products from every cell in the circulation of blood through the capillaries. The capillary walls are so constructed that substances of various molecular sizes can penetrate the surrounding tissue from inside the capillary and also pass into the capillary from the surrounding tissue. Ordinary capillaries are generally regarded as thin-walled tubes consisting of endothelial cells which are joined at their edges. Capillaries are also composed of basement membranes and pericytes.

5.2 Flow of plasma through capillaries

(a) Starling's hypothesis

According to Starling's hypothesis, the filtration and absorption of water across the capillary walls depends upon the net effect of the following four independent factors: (i) hydrostatic capillary blood pressure p_c; (ii) osmotic pressure of plasma proteins π_c; (iii) hydrostatic interstitial fluid pressure p_i, immediately outside the capillary walls; (iv) osmotic pressure π_i of the proteins in the interstitial fluid.

His hypothesis is usually expressed as follows:

$$m = k(p_c - \pi_c - p_i + \pi_i) \tag{5.1}$$

Here m represents the flow rate per unit area of wall surface, with a plus sign to indicate filtration and a minus sign to indicate absorption. The constant k is a measure of the permeability of the capillary wall to water, and it is called the *filtration constant*. The measured value of k is usually expressed in units of cm (s cm H_2O)$^{-1}$. If m stands for the rate of fluid mass movement across the wall of the capillary per unit area, then k is expressed in the units s cm^{-1}. Equation (5.1) indicates that the filtration is proportional to the difference between the quantities $(p_c - \pi_c)$ and $(p_i - \pi_i)$. Filtrated water which passes into the tissues is either reabsorbed into the capillary blood or returned to the blood via the lymphatic system.

It should be pointed out that there is some ambiguity about Eq. (5.1). If the quantity m is defined as the flow rate per unit area of the total wall surface, then p_c cannot vary along the length of the capillary. In this case p_c should be replaced by an appropriate value. If we regard p_c as a local hydrostatic capillary blood pressure, then p_c varies along the length of the capillary, and m should also be considered as the flow rate per unit area of an infinitesimal wall surface. From a theoretical standpoint, the latter view is preferred.

(b) Assumptions and results

In order to analyse theoretically the plasma flow within

5.2 Flow of plasma through capillaries

a capillary as well as the net water exchange per unit time across the capillary wall, the following simplifying assumptions have been made: (i) the capillary is a straight rigid tube of uniform circular cross-section; (ii) plasma is a homogeneous incompressible Newtonian fluid; (iii) the effect of gravity is neglected; (iv) the motion of the fluid is laminar and steady; (v) the motion of the fluid is so slow that the inertia terms can be neglected; (vi) the motion has an axial symmetry; (vii) the capillary is so long that the end-effect can be neglected; (viii) there is no slip at the wall; (ix) the water exchange obeys Starling's hypothesis; (x) the flow rate per unit area of the wall surface is very small; (xi) p_i, π_c, and π_i are all constant; (xii) the filtration constant k is uniform along the length of the capillary.

We shall describe our results briefly (Oka & Murata, 1970):
(1) The centerline axial velocity becomes minimum at $\xi_1 = \Delta\alpha/\Delta p$, where ξ_1 is the normalized axial distance from the arteriolar end of the capillary. $\Delta\alpha$ and Δp are defined by

$$\Delta\alpha = p_a - \alpha \qquad \Delta p = p_a - p_v$$
$$\alpha = p_i + \pi_c - \pi_i \tag{5.2}$$

Here p_a and p_v are, respectively, the arteriolar and venular pressure. The profiles of the axial velocity u and the radial velocity v and the streamlines are shown schematically in Fig. 44.
(2) The flow rate Q, i.e. the volume of the fluid flowing per unit time across the cross-section, is shown in Fig. 45 for three cases. It can be seen that Q reaches a minimum at $\xi_1 = \Delta\alpha/\Delta p$.
(3) The net outflow M of water into the tissue per unit time across the whole capillary surface S is given by

$$M = kS\left(\frac{\Delta\alpha}{\Delta p} - \frac{1}{2}\right) = kS(p_m - \alpha) \tag{5.3}$$

where p_m is the arithmetical mean of p_a and p_v. Thus, we have

$$m' = M/S = k(p_m - \pi_c - p_i + \pi_i) \tag{5.4}$$

where m' is the net outflow of water per unit time averaged over the whole surface area of the capillary. Note that p_c in Eq. (5.1) is replaced by p_m.

(c) Theoretical treatment

Let us take a cylindrical coordinate system (r, ϕ, z). From assumption (ii) above, the fundamental equations are the Navier–Stokes equation and the equation of continuity, which determine u, v and the pressure, p. The boundary conditions are as follows: from assumption (vi) we get $\partial u/\partial r = 0$ at $r = 0$, and also $v = 0$ at $r = 0$. From assumption (viii) we get $u = 0$ at $r = R$. Starling's hypothesis is written in the local form $v = k(p - \alpha)$ at $r = R$. From assumption (xi), α is regarded as constant. The boundary conditions at $z = 0$ and $z = L$ are respectively written as $\bar{p} = p_a$ and $\bar{p} = p_v$, where $\bar{p}$ indicates the average of the pressure p over the cross-section of the capillary. Both p_a and p_v are regarded as constant.

Let us introduce the dimensionless parameter

$$\varepsilon = k\eta/R \tag{5.5}$$

where η is the viscosity of plasma. The average filtration constant is 2.5×10^{-8} cm (s cm H_2O)$^{-1}$ for muscle capillaries of the dog and cat. If we take $\eta = 1$ cP and $R = 5$ μm, then we get $\varepsilon = 1 \times 10^{-7}$. Hence ε may be regarded as very small.

Let us further introduce, for simplicity, the dimensionless parameters

$$\beta = R/L \qquad \zeta = r/R \qquad \xi_1 = z/L \tag{5.6}$$

where ζ is the normalized radial distance from the axis of the capillary. Neglecting small terms of order ε^2 and the higher we get the following approximate solutions:

$$u = \frac{R^2}{4\eta}\frac{\Delta p}{L}(1 - \zeta^2)[1 + \varepsilon f(\zeta, \xi_1)] \tag{5.7}$$

$$v = \frac{\varepsilon R}{\eta}\frac{\Delta p}{L}(2\zeta - \zeta^3)\left(\frac{\Delta \alpha}{\Delta p} - \xi_1\right) \tag{5.8}$$

$$p = p_a - \xi_1 \Delta p + \varepsilon g(\zeta, \xi_1)\Delta p \tag{5.9}$$

with

$$f(\zeta, \xi_1) = \frac{8}{\beta^2}\left[\left(\xi_1 - \frac{\Delta \alpha}{\Delta p}\right)^2 - \left(\frac{\Delta \alpha}{\Delta p}\right)^2 + \frac{\Delta \alpha}{\Delta p} - \frac{1}{3}\right.$$
$$\left. + \frac{1}{2}\beta^2 - \frac{1}{4}\beta^2\zeta^2\right] \tag{5.10}$$

5.2 Flow of plasma through capillaries

$$g(\zeta, \xi_1) = -\frac{8}{3\beta^2}\left[\xi_1^3 - 3\frac{\Delta\alpha}{\Delta p}\xi_1^2 \right.$$
$$\left. - \left\{1 - 3\frac{\Delta\alpha}{\Delta p} - \frac{3}{4}\beta^2(1 - 2\zeta^2)\right\}\xi_1 \right.$$
$$\left. - \frac{3}{4}\beta^2\frac{\Delta\alpha}{\Delta p}(1 - 2\zeta^2) \right] \quad (5.11)$$

Note that Eqs. (5.7)–(5.9) are reduced to the familiar formulas for the Poiseuille flow in the limit $k \to 0$, i.e. $\varepsilon \to 0$.

Equation (5.7) indicates that the profile of axial velocity u at any cross-section ξ_1 is not strictly parabolic, the deviation from the

Fig. 44. Velocity profiles and streamlines of plasma through a capillary with a permeable wall. (From Oka & Murata, 1970.)

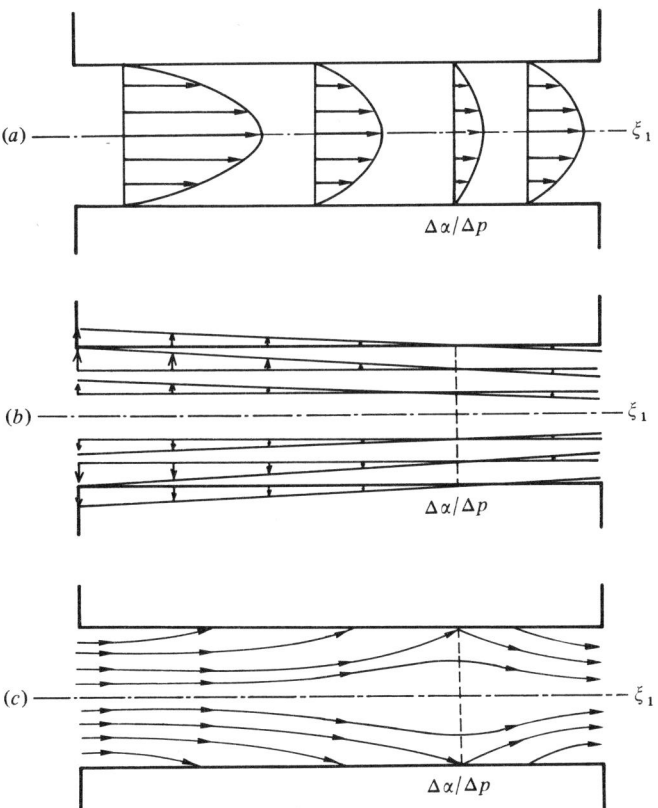

parabolic distribution being of the order of ε. The velocity u reaches a maximum at the axis. The centerline velocity reaches a minimum at the point $\xi_1 = \Delta\alpha/\Delta p$, while it decreases or increases with ξ_1 in the region $\xi_1 < \Delta\alpha/\Delta p$ or $\xi_1 > \Delta\alpha/\Delta p$, respectively. The centerline velocity increases or decreases with ξ_1 depending on whether $\Delta\alpha/\Delta p < 1$ or $\Delta\alpha/\Delta p > 1$, respectively. Figure 44(a) shows the velocity profile u schematically for the case $0 < \Delta\alpha/\Delta p < 1$.

Figure 44(b) indicates that the radial velocity v varies linearly with ξ_1 and vanishes at the point $\xi_1 = \Delta\alpha/\Delta p$. v is positive or negative depending on whether $\xi_1 < \Delta\alpha/\Delta p$ or $\xi_1 > \Delta\alpha/\Delta p$, respectively. Since the radial velocity at the wall is given by

$$v(1,\xi_1) = \frac{\varepsilon R}{\eta}\left(\frac{\Delta\alpha}{\Delta p} - \xi_1\right) \tag{5.12}$$

outflow and inflow appear in the regions $\xi_1 < \Delta\alpha/\Delta p$ and $\xi_1 > \Delta\alpha/\Delta p$, respectively. Figure 44 considers the case $0 < \Delta\alpha/\Delta p < 1$. When $\Delta\alpha/\Delta p = \frac{1}{2}$, the outflow and inflow are balanced. When $\Delta\alpha/\Delta p < 0$, i.e. $p_a < \alpha$, we have only inflow along the entire length of the capillary. Similarly, only outflow appears in the case where $\Delta\alpha/\Delta p > 1$, i.e. $p_v > \alpha$. These cases can actually be observed in microcirculation. The streamlines are schematically shown in Fig. 44(c).

From Eq. (5.9) it can be seen that the pressure does not change in a strictly linear fashion with the distance z.

The flow rate Q is calculated from Eq. (2.18). By use of Eqs. (5.7) and (5.10) we obtain

$$Q = \frac{\pi R^4}{8\eta}\frac{\Delta p}{L}\left[1 + \varepsilon f\left(\frac{1}{\sqrt{3}}, \xi_1\right)\right] \tag{5.13}$$

which is reduced to Poiseuille's law when k tends to zero.

Since $f(1/\sqrt{3},\xi_1)$ reaches a minimum at $\xi_1 = \Delta\alpha/\Delta p$, Q also reaches a minimum at $\xi_1 = \Delta\alpha/\Delta p$. The relationship between Q and ξ_1 is shown schematically in Fig. 45. The decrease of the flow rate with increase in ξ_1 in the region $0 < \xi_1 < \Delta\alpha/\Delta p$ is caused by filtration, and the increase of the flow rate with ξ_1 in the region $\Delta\alpha/\Delta p < \xi_1 < 1$ is caused by absorption.

The net outflow M or water into the tissue per unit time across the capillary wall can be calculated by $M = Q(0) - Q(1)$. By use of

5.2 Flow of plasma through capillaries

Eqs. (5.13) and (5.10) we have

$$M = \varepsilon \frac{2\pi R^4}{\eta \beta^2} \frac{\Delta p}{L}\left(\frac{\Delta \alpha}{\Delta p} - \frac{1}{2}\right) = kS\left(\frac{\Delta \alpha}{\Delta p} - \frac{1}{2}\right) \qquad (5.14)$$

When $\Delta \alpha/\Delta p = \frac{1}{2}$, $M = 0$, i.e. outflow and inflow are balanced. When $\Delta \alpha/\Delta p > \frac{1}{2}$, $M > 0$, we have no outflow, while for $\Delta \alpha/\Delta p < \frac{1}{2}$, we have no inflow.

It is interesting that Eq. (5.14) can be derived in another way. The net outflow can also be calculated from the radial component v at the wall. It is found to be identical with Eq. (5.14) by using Eq. (5.12).

This fact may be regarded as varifying our solutions to Eqs. (5.7)–(5.9).

In the above theory, it is assumed that a capillary is a straight tube of uniform circular cross-section. But capillaries are actually curved and branched. The blood flow through a capillary is so slow that the Reynolds number becomes $Re = 0.0007$–0.003, and hence the effect of inertia is negligible compared with that of viscosity. It has been pointed out by Lighthill (1969) that the effect of curvature can be neglected in this case. Hence, the assumption of a straight tube may be allowed.

In the above theory, both the quantities α and k are regarded as constant. In the case of edema, α may depend upon the time and also possibly upon the position. It is not yet clear experimentally how k varies along the length of the capillary. Although many experiments have looked at the dependence of the filtration of various dyestuffs on the position of microvessels, it is hard to judge

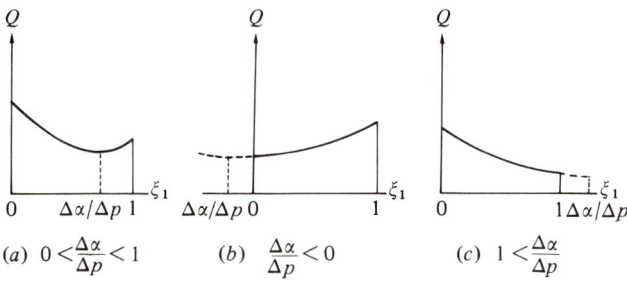

Fig. 45. Three cases of flow rate vs. axial distance.

(a) $0 < \frac{\Delta \alpha}{\Delta p} < 1$ (b) $\frac{\Delta \alpha}{\Delta p} < 0$ (c) $1 < \frac{\Delta \alpha}{\Delta p}$

the filtration of water from the data concerning the filtration of dyestuffs, due to differences in molecular size. They may also use different pathways through the walls.

(d) Occluded capillary

In order to confirm Starling's hypothesis, Landis (1927) introduced micropipettes into the lumen of capillaries and determined the pressure within them. He occluded the capillary by a microscopic rod so that fluid movement could only be due to escape through the walls, and estimated the rate of fluid movement by the rate at which a red cell moved towards or away from the blocked end.

Lew & Fung (1969b) did a theoretical study of the motion of

Fig. 46. Velocity profiles of plasma flow in an occluded capillary. (From Lew & Fung, 1969b.)

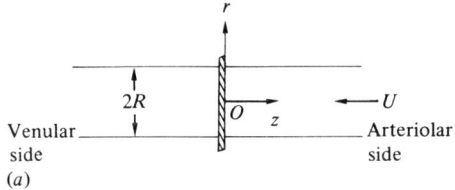

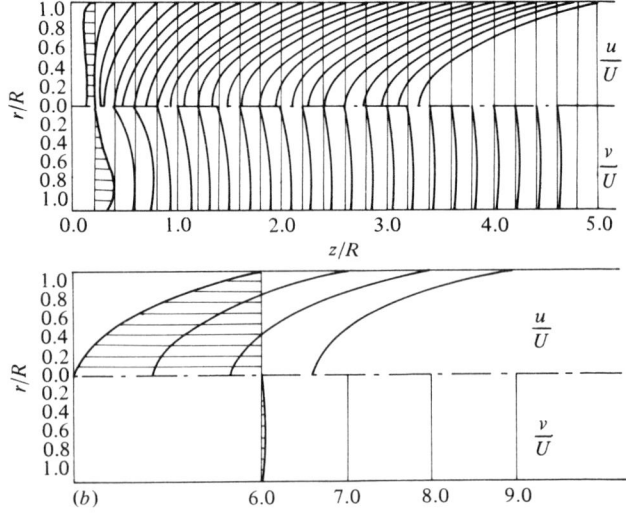

plasma in a capillary blood vessel which is occluded at one point (Fig. 46(a)). A capillary blood vessel is suddenly occluded at O. It is assumed that the dimensions and conditions in the arteriole, venule, and the tissue surrounding the capillary are unaffected by the occlusion. Before occlusion, the system is assumed to be in a steady state. After occlusion, the osmotic pressures both inside and outside the capillary are assumed to remain constant. The effect of the presence of red blood cells is not taken into account. The no-slip condition of the fluid at the wall is also assumed. For the boundary conditions upstream it is assumed that the tube is so long that the upstream condition may be replaced by a condition at infinity.

Numerical calculations were performed for the case of long tubes. Figure 46(b) shows the velocity profiles of flow in an occluded capillary when the parameter $k\eta/R$ is 0.01. The upper half of each figure shows the distribution of the normalized axial velocity component u/U as a function of the radial coordinate r at points $z/R = 0$, $0.2, 0.4, \ldots, 9.0$. The lower half of each figure shows the corresponding distribution of the normalized radial velocity component v/U. It should be noted that the radial velocity is not maximum at the wall. For a capillary which is not occluded, our theory suggests that the radial velocity distribution obeys $2(r/R) - (r/R)^3$, i.e. the radial velocity is maximum at $r/R = \sqrt{2/3} = 0.816$.

5.3 Flow of Casson fluid through a capillary

The preceding section only considered the flow of a Newtonian fluid, since the theory was based on the Navier–Stokes equation. This section extends our theory of the flow of a Casson fluid through a capillary with permeable walls (Oka, 1979).

The pressure–flow relationship for the flow of a Casson fluid in a small tube with a non-permeable wall has already been obtained theoretically by the present writer in the form

$$Q = \frac{\pi R^4}{8\eta_C} \frac{\Delta p}{L} F(\xi) \qquad [(3.18)]$$

where R is the inner radius, L is the length of the tube, and Δp is the pressure difference between the ends of the tube. The Casson fluid is specified by the Casson viscosity η_C and the Casson yield stress f_C. The function $F(\xi)$ is given by Eq. (3.19), and ξ is a dimensionless quantity defined by Eq. (3.20), i.e.

$$\xi = 2f_C L/R\Delta p \tag{5.15}$$

We shall now consider the combined effect of permeability of the capillary wall and the non-Newtonian behavior of blood. Let the flow rate at any point ξ_1 of a capillary be denoted by $Q(\xi_1; k, f_C)$, where k and f_C are parameters. They are small quantities. For instance, k is 2.5×10^{-8} cm (s cm H_2O)$^{-1}$ for muscle capillaries of the dog and cat as mentioned before, and f_C is approximately 0.2 dyn cm^{-2} for human blood of Ht 45%.

Let us expand $Q(\xi_1; k, f_C)$ in the neighborhood of $k = 0$ and $f_C = 0$. We retain the first order term in k, neglecting small terms of the second and higher orders in k. As is seen from Eqs. (3.18), (3.19) and (5.15), $Q(\xi_1; 0, f_C)$ contains only terms of orders $\sqrt{f_C}, f_C$ and f_C^4, so that we may write

$$Q(\xi_1; k, f_C) = Q(\xi_1; 0, 0) + kQ_1 + \sqrt{f_C}Q_2$$
$$+ f_C Q_3 + f_C^4 Q_4 \tag{5.16}$$

where Q_1, Q_2, Q_3, and Q_4 are constants to be determined. Since Eq. (5.16) should become identical with Eq. (3.18) in the limit $k \to 0$, we can obtain $Q(\xi_1; 0, 0)$, Q_2, Q_3 and Q_4. In the case of the limit $f_C \to 0$, the Casson fluid should become a Newtonian fluid with the viscosity η_C. Then, considering Eq. (5.16) in the limit $f \to 0$, we have Q_1 from Eq. (13). Substitution of these values into Eq. (5.16) gives the final result:

$$Q(\xi_1; k, f_C) = \frac{\pi R^4}{8\eta_C} \frac{\Delta p}{L} F(\xi) + \frac{\pi R^4}{8} \frac{k}{R} f\left(\frac{1}{\sqrt{3}}, \xi_1\right) \tag{5.17}$$

The first term depends on the yield stress as well as the viscosity, but not on the permeability. This may be called the non-Newtonian term. The second term depends on the permeability, but not on the yield stress or the viscosity. This may be called the permeability term.

The net outflow of water, M, into the tissue is given by

$$M = Q(\xi_1; k, f_C)|_{\xi_1 = 0} - Q(\xi_1; k, f_C)|_{\xi_1 = 1}$$

5.3 Flow of Casson fluid through a capillary

or

$$M = \frac{\pi R^4}{8} \frac{\Delta p}{L} \left[\frac{F(\xi)}{\eta_C} \bigg|_{\xi_1 = 0} - \frac{F(\xi)}{\eta_C} \bigg|_{\xi_1 = 1} \right] + kS \left(\frac{\Delta \alpha}{\Delta p} - \frac{1}{2} \right) \tag{5.18}$$

where S is the whole surface area of the capillary. The second term was obtained in Eq. (5.14). It should be noted that the first term will not vanish in general, because both the Casson yield stress and the Casson viscosity are influenced by the change of hematocrit, which is caused by the filtration and absorption of water.

The effect of hematocrit on the Casson yield stress was described in Chapter 3. Various empirical formulas have been suggested for the relationship between the apparent viscosity η_a of blood and the hematocrit, but little is yet known about the relationship between the Casson viscosity η_C and the hematocrit. An empirical formula was recently proposed by Shiga et al. (1979):

$$\ln (\eta_C/\eta_p) = \text{const } H \qquad [(3.9)]$$

where η_p is the viscosity of plasma and H is the hematocrit.

If we compare Eq. (5.17) with Eq. (5.13), the effect of non-Newtonian behavior of blood can be seen in the function $F(\xi)$ instead of unity. The value of $F(\xi)$ depends, of course, on the value of R, L, Δp and f_C, and the value of f_C depends not only on the hematocrit, but also on the method of measurement. If we choose $R = 5\mu\text{m}$, $L = 300\,\mu\text{m}$, $\Delta p = 17$ mm Hg, then we have $\xi = 0.00529 f_C$. Several values of ξ and $F(\xi)$ are given in Table 2. It is clear that the flow rate of blood is greatly influenced by the Casson yield stress. It is also clear that the usual formula for the net outflow of water should be modified by taking into account the non-Newtonian behavior of blood.

Table 2. $F(\xi)$ vs. ξ.

f_C(dyn cm^{-2})	ξ	$F(\xi)$
0.01	0.000	0.99
0.2	0.001	0.93
5	0.027	0.66
10	0.053	0.55

5.4 Capillary–tissue fluid exchange

So far we have limited ourselves to the flow of fluid within a capillary, without taking into account the flow through the tissue region.

The first theoretical study on the exchange of oxygen across the capillary walls and the tissue surrounding them was made by Krogh (1919). He observed in detail the distribution of capillaries in muscle, and proposed a functional unit of capillary beds. *Krogh's model* is composed of a long straight cylindrical capillary and a concentric cylinder of homogeneous tissue surrounding it (Fig. 47).

With regard to the validity of Starling's hypothesis, Wiederhielm (1968) drew, after careful experimental examination, the following conclusions: (i) the filtration constant may be 50 to 100% larger in the venous capillary than in the arterial capillary; (ii) the surface area of the arterial capillaries may be only $\frac{1}{6}$ to $\frac{1}{4}$ of that of the venous capillaries; (iii) the hydrostatic and osmotic pressures of interstitial fluid are not negligible compared with the corresponding blood values; (iv) the average value of the osmotic pressure of interstitial fluid is 5 to 8 mm Hg referred to the atmospheric pressure; (v) the hydrostatic interstitial fluid pressures range from 0 to 5 mm Hg by direct measurements, whereas pressures recorded in subcutaneous capsules are negative and average -6 mm Hg.

Apelblat, Katchalsky & Silberberg (1974) studied the capillary–tissue fluid exchange theoretically from various points of view. Their treatment was based on Krogh's model. Within the capillary the Navier–Stokes equation and the equation of continuity were solved approximately. The tissue regions were treated as isotropic porous media to which Darcy's law is applicable. Since the no-slip

Fig. 47. Krogh's model.

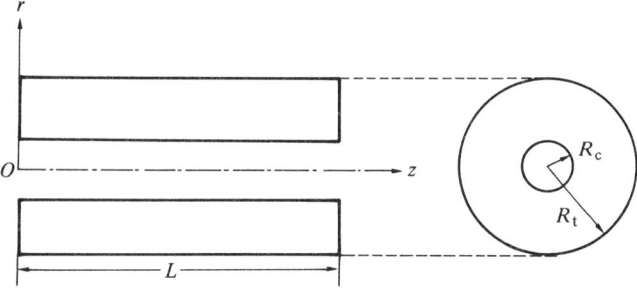

5.4 Capillary–tissue fluid exchange

condition at the capillary wall in the tissue region was not satisfied, the condition for the tangential component of velocity at the capillary wall in the tissue region was left unspecified. In this model it was assumed that the filtration constant was uniform and that there was no lymph flow.

Darcy's law states that the flow is directly proportional to the applied pressure gradient:

$$\mathbf{v} = -\frac{K}{\eta}\nabla p \qquad (5.19)$$

where $\mathbf{v}$ is the velocity vector, and ∇ represents the gradient. In the above, $\mathbf{v}$ is averaged over a tissue volume which is large compared with the volume of an individual pore. η is the viscosity of plasma, and K is *Darcy's constant*, which characterizes the porosity of the medium.

Apelblat *et al.* analysed filtration from a cylindrical capillary into a concentrically surrounding tissue space; flow from a capillary into the tissue across a thin membrane; filtration from a rectangular, a cylindrical and a conical channel bounded by a permeable material of uniform or regionally different permeability; and transcapillary fluid exchange. For biological systems which are characterized by low permeability, the calculations show that any factor which produces a nonlinear distribution of pressure in the capillary will increase the filtration efficiency per unit of permeable area. Nonlinear pressure distribution arises, for example, due to an asymmetry of geometrical structure or due to the interaction between the red blood cell and wall during cell movement down the capillary. It is shown that thin membranes of low permeability on a sufficiently thick layer of tissue reduce the pressure gradient in the tissue to a very small value compared with the pressure gradient of blood flow in the capillary.

The characteristic feature of flow in the tissue region is that its velocity decreases markedly in the layer of 2–3 capillary radii around the cylinder. Distribution of pressure in the high pressure half of Krogh's model is shown in Fig. 48. The streamlines and the isobars form an orthogonal net of curves. It can be seen that the tissue is mostly under an axial pressure gradient, indicating that the flow is mainly parallel to the capillary axis.

An & Salathe (1976) showed that large gradients of interstitial fluid pressure normal to the capillary wall occur in the tissue spaces adjacent to the capillary wall. They showed that these gradients have a significant effect on fluid exchange, so that the assumption of uniform distribution of interstitial fluid pressure cannot be accepted. They considered a straight circular capillary with variable radius surrounded by a tissue space of infinite extent, the fluid exchange between the capillary and the surrounding tissue being governed by Starling's law. They assumed that the flow within the capillary is governed by Poiseuille's law and that

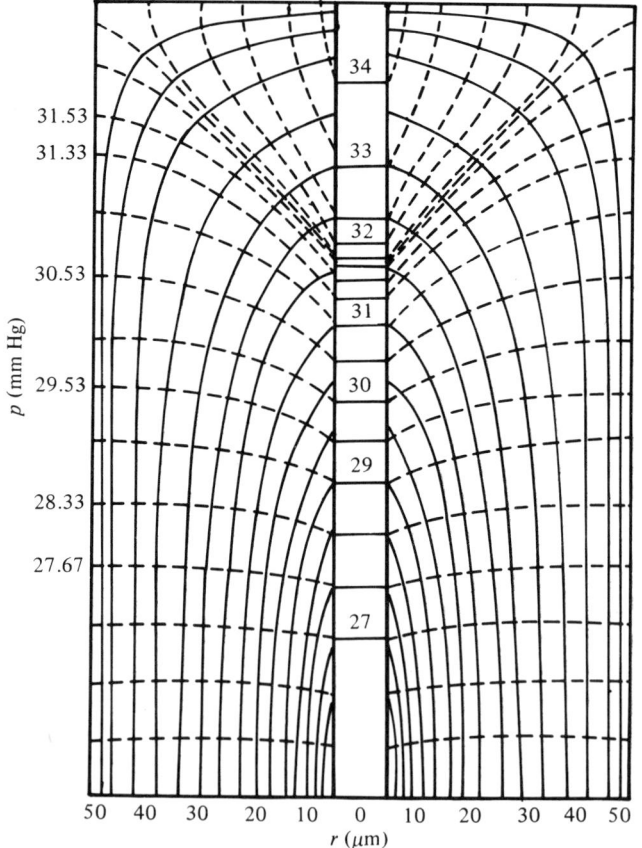

Fig. 48. Streamlines and pressure distribution in a Krogh's model. (From Apelblat et al., 1974.)

5.4 Capillary–tissue fluid exchange

the flow within the tissue is governed by Darcy's law. Assuming that the ratio of radius to length of the capillary is very small and that the filtration constant is very small, they obtained an approximate solution of the pressure allowing for arbitrary variation of capillary radius and permeability. Numerical results were also obtained when the radius and the filtration constant k vary in a linear fashion. However, the tangential component of the velocity at the capillary wall in the tissue space did not satisfy the no-slip condition because of the use of Darcy's law. They also neglected the effect of flow of fluid from the tissue space to the lymphatic capillaries on the pressure distributions.

Murata (1978) analysed theoretically the effects of variable filtration constant, k, and lymph flow on fluid exchange between the blood capillary and the tissue space, using Krogh's model and Starling's law. He assumed that the filtration constant of the capillary wall was not uniform along the length of capillary, but increases linearly with the distance from the arterial end. He further assumed that the flow of fluid through the tissue region was governed by a *generalized Darcy's law* derived theoretically by Tam (1969). Under these assumptions, the velocity and pressure distributions in the capillary and tissue regions were obtained. The average interstitial fluid

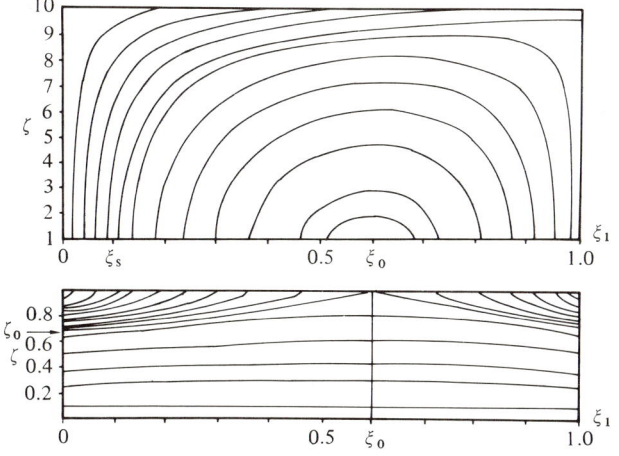

Fig. 49. Streamlines within a capillary and tissue region. (From Murata, 1978.)

pressure and the average effective pressure difference between the blood and interstitial fluid were also obtained.

Since the lymphatic capillary networks are distributed through the interstitial spaces along with the blood capillaries, the terminal vessels of the two systems must lie very near each other. The lymphatic capillaries are commonly believed to end blindly in interstitial spaces at varying distances from the blood capillaries. In order to introduce the lymphatic capillaries into Krogh's model without destroying its axial symmetry, he assumed that the lymphatic capillaries were distributed uniformly on the outer surface of the tissue region of Krogh's model. He further assumed that the fluid entered into the lymphatic capillary with a constant velocity from the outer surface of the tissue region of Krogh's model, and that the lymph flow was proportional to the filtration rate.

Tam derived the generalized Darcy's law when fluid flows very slowly through a porous medium consisting of small spherical particles. This is expressed as:

$$\nabla p = \eta(\nabla^2 \mathbf{v} - \sigma^2 \mathbf{v}) \tag{5.20}$$

where ∇ stands for Laplacian operator. σ^2 represents the flow resistance; it depends upon the particle size as well as the volume concentration of particles. Note that Eq. (5.20) is reduced to Darcy's original law, Eq. (5.19), when σ^2 is very large. Then the Darcy constant K in Eq. (5.19) corresponds to $1/\sigma^2$.

The streamlines are shown in Fig. 49 for a given set of parameters. The fluid transferred into the tissue region across the capillary wall over the range $0 < \xi < \xi_s$ flows into the lymphatic capillaries across the outer surface of the tissue, and the fluid entering the capillary over the range $\xi_0 < \xi < 1$ flows into the tissue region across the capillary wall.

5.5 Bolus flow

The blood flow in capillaries is characterized by the fact that their diameters approach the size of the red blood cell. Then the red cells move either alone or in groups, separated axially by plasmatic gaps. This type of blood flow is referred to as 'bolus flow' or sometimes as 'axial-train flow'. The first observation of the particulate nature of blood was made by Leeuwenhoek (1688) in a

5.5 Bolus flow

capillary of the tail of a fish. Later observation of the capillary beds of the microcirculation showed that the red cells tend to follow each other axially in single file with their discoidal surfaces roughly perpendicular to the axis of the capillary (Fig. 50). Note that the eddy motion is shown relative to the red cells.

Prothero & Burton (1962) were the first to perform experiments with a large scale physical model, consisting of a train of air bubbles separated by water flowing through a cylindrical tube. The air bubbles simulate the red blood cells. They injected dyes into the water and observed an eddy motion which circulated the water in the gaps between the bubbles. The eddy motion was found to increase as the dimensions of the water in the gaps between the air bubbles decreased. Based on the model experiments, they suggested that the eddy motion in the plasmatic gaps between red blood cells in the blood flow through a capillary was important. Thus, the eddy motion was considered to be responsible for the energy dissipation and the mass (oxygen) and heat transfer taking place in the capillary.

It is questionable, however, whether Prothero & Burton's experiments are applicable to capillary flow, because their experiments were performed at Reynolds numbers of the order of 10 and higher, whereas the Reynolds numbers of typical capillary flows are of the order of 0.01 and less. The eddy motion associated with bolus flow would be much less effective in mixing the plasma between red cells because of the negligible inertial effect.

Since it is difficult to measure directly the eddy motion in the plasmatic gaps, owing to the small lumen of the capillary, theoretical

Fig. 50. Bolus flow relative to the red cells. (From Whitmore, 1968.)

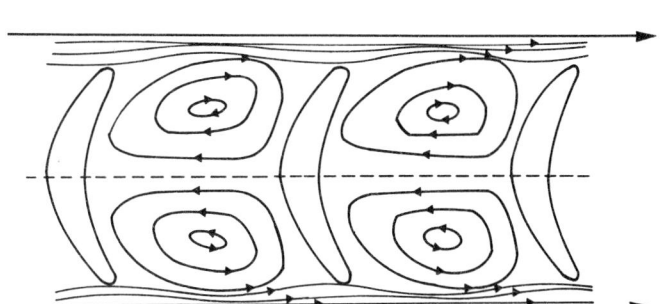

analyses of bolus flow have been put forward by many investigators based on various mathematical models.

For example, Wang & Skalak (1969) considered a model containing a train of rigid spheres in a rigid tube. Streamlines and velocity profiles are shown in Fig. 51.

On the other hand, Lew & Fung (1969a) considered a different model, containing cylindrical pill boxes whose radii are equal to that of the rigid tube. Velocity and pressure profiles between two 'cells' moving slowly through a capillary were solved analytically for very low Reynolds numbers.

In Fig. 52 the mean pressure gradient $\partial \langle p \rangle / \partial z$ is plotted vs. $2L/R$ to show how the effective viscosity varies with the hematocrit, which is related to the intercellular distance. $\langle p \rangle$ is the pressure averaged over the cross-section of the capillary. Thus, resistance to flow through a capillary is increased by the presence of closely spaced red cells, due to the eddy motion in the plasmatic gaps.

If there is a small clearance between the capillary wall and the red cells, a pressure loss will be added due to the high shear rates

Fig. 51. Bolus flow of rigid spheres. (a) relative to the tube, i.e. spheres are moving, (b) relative to the spheres, i.e. observer is moving with spheres so that they appear fixed and walls move backwards. (From Wang & Skalak, 1969.)

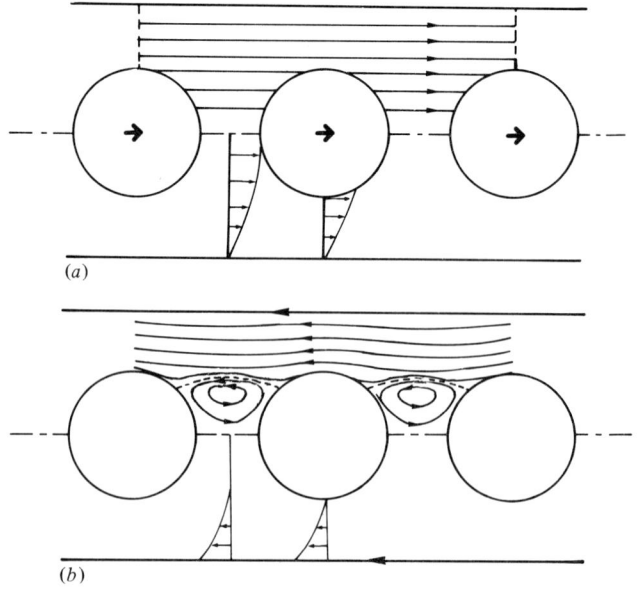

5.5 Bolus flow

within the clearance. If the red cell is larger than the capillary, both the red cell and capillary wall will deform so that the red cell does not necessarily contact the capillary wall.

Bugliarello & Hsiao (1970) studied the flow in the plasmatic gaps of the capillaries of the microcirculation for three axisymmetric models: red blood cells spanning the entire lumen, with red cell–plasma interface straight (model A) and curved (model B), and red cells spanning only a portion of the lumen, with straight interface (model C). Model A is the same as that of Lew & Fung. The most important finding is that the circulation in the plasmatic gaps is of primary importance in determining the pressure drop, but contrary to Prothero & Burton's suggestion, it can have only limited influence on the oxygen and heat transfer processes in a capillary.

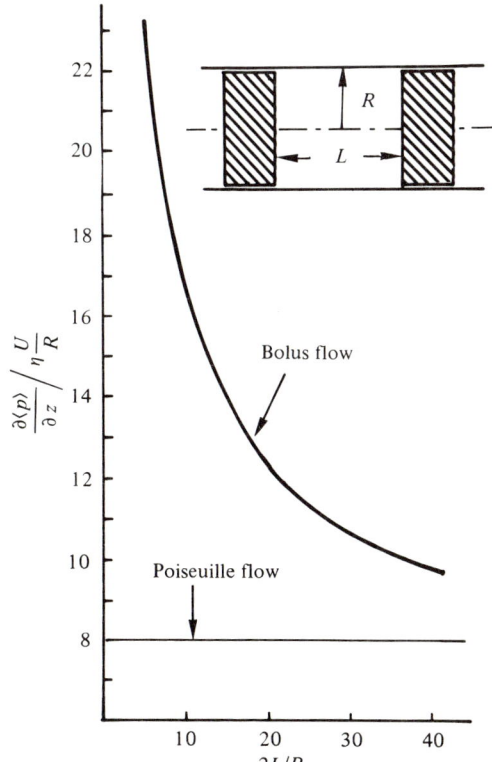

Fig. 52. Bolus flow of cylindrical pill boxes. (From Lew & Fung, 1969.)

Assuming a diffusion coefficient D for oxygen in plasma of 2×10^{-5} cm^2 s^{-1}, and a radius R of capillary of 5 μm, a time of the order of $R^2/2D = 6 \times 10^{-3}$ s is required by oxygen to diffuse to the centerline, in the absence of convective currents. Bugliarello & Hsiao calculated a circulation time which is greater than diffusion time, indicating that circulation is ineffective in enhancing mass transfer. With physiologically representative conditions, the circulation time would be of the order of 10^{-1} s, two orders of magnitude larger than the diffusion time. Duda & Vrentas (1971) arrived at the same conclusions quantitatively by use of the Péclet number, UR/D.

Skalak, Chen & Chien (1972) considered a model of capillary blood flow consisting of red-cell shaped particles suspended in a Newtonian fluid. They assumed that the red cells were axisymmetrically located in a circular tube with their discoidal surfaces perpendicular to the axis of the tube. They assumed that red cells maintained their biconcave disc shape during the motion. The cells are equally spaced along the tube and the motion is assumed to be sufficiently slow to make inertial terms negligible.

They applied the finite element method to the flow of plasmatic gaps to determine the effect of hematocrit and rouleaux on apparent viscosity in capillaries. They showed that the apparent viscosity varies linearly with hematocrit at low hematocrits. This is due to the fact that widely spaced cells do not interact, and the pressure drop is then proportional to the number of cells per unit length, which varies directly with the hematocrit. However, the apparent viscosity increases less rapidly at high hematocrits. This is due to the fact that at small cell spacings the fluid between cells is more or less immobilized. The effect of rouleaux is to decrease slightly the apparent viscosity at fixed hematocrit. The effect is largest at low hematocrits, which corresponds to wide spacings. At higher hematocrits, the fluid is immobilized between adjacent cells and the formation of rouleaux then has less effect.

5.6 Sheet flow

The capillaries in the pulmonary alveoli are so short and so closely knit that it may be better to discard the usual notion of a blood vessel as a tube. Weibel (1962), from an extensive morpho-

5.6 Sheet flow

metric study of the human lung, proposed an idealized geometric model. The *Weibel model* consists of a hexagonal network of short, circular cylindrical tubes (Fig. 53). Weibel showed that the tube length a and the tube diameter d are of the same order of magnitude, and used the word 'sheet' to describe the capillary blood vessel network in the pulmonary alveoli. The number of such sheets in a human lung is of the order of 10^9.

The Weibel model was simplified by rounding off the corners of the hexagonal posts and smoothing off the wrinkles at the top and bottom. The alveolar sheet is then regarded as composed of two flat membranes linked by a number of posts. This model is referred to as the *Sobin–Fung model*, and its main characteristics are the distance between posts, the diameter of the circular cylindrical post, and the sheet thickness. Note that this model is made only for the purpose of studying fluid mechanics. The posts are cells connecting the alveolar cells, and the walls and the posts are thin and flexible structures.

Fig. 53. Weibel's model of alveolar capillaries. (From Weibel, 1962.)

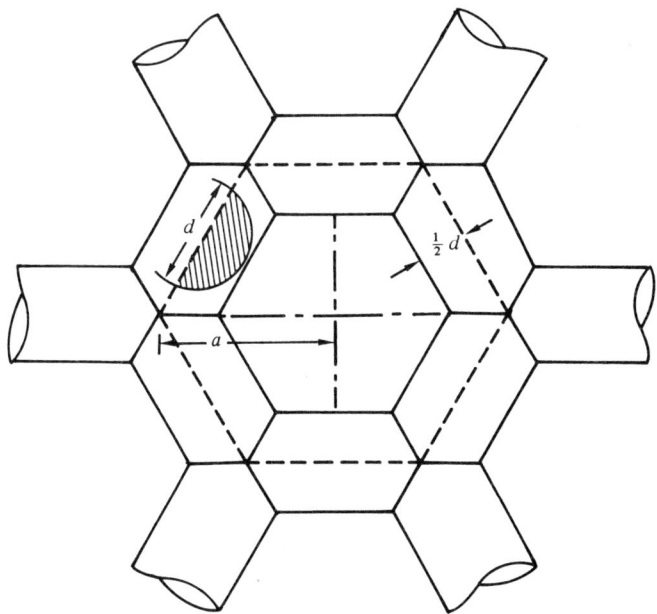

In order to analyse mathematically the blood pressure, velocity distribution, and thickness variation of the pulmonary alveoli sheet, Fung & Sobin (1969) introduced the important concept of the local average of a quantity over a small area covering a number of posts. Similar treatment is generally used in physics when macroscopic quantities are interpreted in terms of microscopic quantities. The local average is denoted by a bar above the quantity. For example, the local average sheet thickness $\bar{h}$ is related to the local average blood pressure $\bar{p}$ by the equation

$$\bar{h} = h_0 + \alpha(\bar{p} - p_A), \tag{5.21}$$

where p_A is the alveolar air pressure, and α is a constant which depends on the tension in the sheet as well as on the elasticity of the posts. Assuming Newtonian viscosity of blood and Hookean elasticity of the sheet, they showed that $\Delta \bar{h}^4 = 0$. The local average pressure and velocity can be obtained under specified boundary conditions.

In relation to the above-mentioned Fung–Sobin theory, a fluid mechanical theory of the flow around a single post confined between two parallel plates was performed by Lee & Fung (1969). Numerical results indicate that the dimensionless resistance of the flow drops rapidly at first and then gradually levels off as the ratio of the distance between two plates to the post diameter increases. Lee (1969) did a further study based on a model consisting of two parallel plates interconnected by regularly spaced circular posts. He concluded that an approximate periodic solution is adequate when the ratio of sheet thickness to post diameter is not much larger than unity.

5.7 Microcirculation and clinical medicine

A number of important clinical changes in microcirculation are associated with shock, low blood pressure, alteration of vascular walls, leukocytosis, platelet thromboembolism, increases in fibrinogen concentration and hematocrit, changes in red cell surface, exposure to cold, altered clotting, changes in vascular permeability, and so on. Hypoxia and metabolic alterations, particularly acidosis, alter red cell membrane elasticity, increase blood viscosity, decrease blood flow, and impair vascular reactivity.

5.7 Microcirculation and clinical medicine

(a) *Microcirculation in diabetes*

One of the most important problems in the pathophysiology of diabetes is the mechanism of microangiopathy, and how to prevent this complication from developing further. It has been pointed out that microangiopathy is caused mainly by insufficient insulin action and morphological and chemical changes in the capillaries, particularly in the glomerulus, retina, muscle, and skin. It has recently been suggested that a possible cause is microcirculatory failure, which in turn results from abnormal viscous flow, intravascular red cell aggregation, hypercoagulability, and low fibrinolytic activity of blood.

There is much evidence suggesting a close relationship between microangiopathy and hemorheology. In fact, in diabetic retinopathy the basement membranes thicken and microaneurysms develop, and stationary blood flow is frequently observed in the capillaries.

Isogai (1976) showed that rheological parameters such as the red cell sedimentation rate, plasma viscosity, blood viscosity, platelet aggregation, plasma fibrinogen, maximum dynamic shear modulus of blood coagulum, and grade of sludging were higher in diabetic patients than in healthy subjects. He also found that, comparing each of these factors, the ratio of the value in diabetic patients to that in healthy subjects was more or less the same.

(b) *Microcirculation in hypoglycemia*

It is now well-known that microcirculation is markedly affected by insulin administration. These effects were first studied by Asano. Later Asano and his coworkers (1975a) studied cutaneous microcirculatory responses to insulin administration in a transparent chamber installed in the ear of a rabbit, which during the experiments was deprived of food, using photomicrography and microphotoelectric plethysmography. They noted that a marked and persistent vasoconstriction and a low-flow state invariably developed with the onset of hypoglycemia. In the slow blood flow, leukocytes showed a strong tendency to adhere, especially to venules; in arterioles they obstructed the flow of red cells into the distal vessels, thus causing a profound microcirculatory hypohematocrit-hypoperfusion. Although leukocytes adhering to venules were not easily washed away, even by the rapid blood flow, they never formed aggregates, thrombi, or coagulates.

Asano *et al.* (1975b) further studied cutaneous microcirculatory responses to insulin administration in the rabbit, which was given hexamethonium bromide (C_6) and deprived of food. C_6-pretreatment caused a long-term dilatation of all blood vessels with an increase in blood flow velocity in the microcirculatory net within the ear chamber. When insulin was given one hour after the C_6, hypoglycemia occurred along with the slower flow of red cells, although the C_6-induced vasodilatation did not subside. When the red cells flowed slowly, leukocytes showed a marked tendency to adhere to all microvessels despite the dilatation. Thus hyperperfusion occurred with plasma but not with red cells; however, adhesive leukocytes never formed aggregates, thrombi, or coagulates.

6

Rheology of blood vessels

6.1 Blood vessel walls

Since Stephen Hales (1733), the importance of vascular distensibility has been recognized, especially for changing the intermittent pumping of the heart into a steady flow in the vein. Rheology of blood vessels has become of great importance for understanding the cardiovascular system.

The rheological properties of blood vessels depend not only on their composition but also on their structure and ultrastructure. Current knowledge about their structure is still at the level of qualitative description. The structure of blood vessels varies along the vascular tree. Structurally, the walls of arteries and veins may be divided into three layers: tunica intima or interna, tunica media, and tunica adventitia or externa. The layers are usually referred to as the intima, media, and adventia, respectively. All arteries and veins are lined by a layer of flattened endothelial cells (endothelium). Other elements of their walls include smooth muscle cells, collagen, elastin, basement membranes, connective tissue, microfibrils, fibrocytes, and other relatively undifferentiated cells. Although arteries and veins are composed of the same cellular and non-cellular connective tissues, there are distinct architectural differences.

In general, there are two main types of artery: the elastic and muscular. Elastic arteries are those closest to the heart, including the aorta, innominate, subclavian, the common carotid, and the main pulmonary arteries. Arteries of muscular type comprise the majority of the distal arteries, and are called the distributing arteries. The type of artery is not dependent on caliber. The architecture is dependent on the position in each animal species. Figure 54 shows a useful summary of the range of size of lumen, thickness of the wall, and composition of the wall in terms of important types of tissues. Hereafter, we limit ourselves mainly to large blood vessels.

The mechanical properties and structure of blood vessels are very complicated, but blood vessels may be treated approximately as hollow cylindrical tubes composed of homogeneous isotropic Hookean solids. Actually, blood vessels are slightly tapered, the tapering angles being about $1-2°$. The word 'homogeneous' means that mechanical properties are identical in any small volume of the vessel wall. Histologically, a segment of the blood vessel may be considered uniform in the longitudinal and the circumferential directions, but not in the radial direction. Therefore, homogeneity is, strictly speaking, an assumption. The word 'isotropic' means that the blood vessel wall has the same elastic properties in all directions. Actually, the blood vessel wall is elastically anisotropic, and its anisotropy will be discussed in the latter part of this chapter.

The blood vessel wall may be regarded as incompressible. In fact, Bergel (1961) measured Young's modulus E, Poisson's ratio σ, and bulk modulus K in the large arteries of dogs and found $E = 4.3 \times 10^6$ dyn cm^{-2}, $\sigma = 0.499$, $K = 4.35 \times 10^9$ dyn cm^{-2}. One can then find the shear modulus G and the ratio of bulk modulus to shear modulus from Table 1, as follows: $G = 1.4 \times 10^6$ dyn cm^{-2}, $K/G \approx 3000$. The above estimation indicates that the aortic wall is incompressible.

Blood vessels *in situ* are attached to the surrounding tissues.

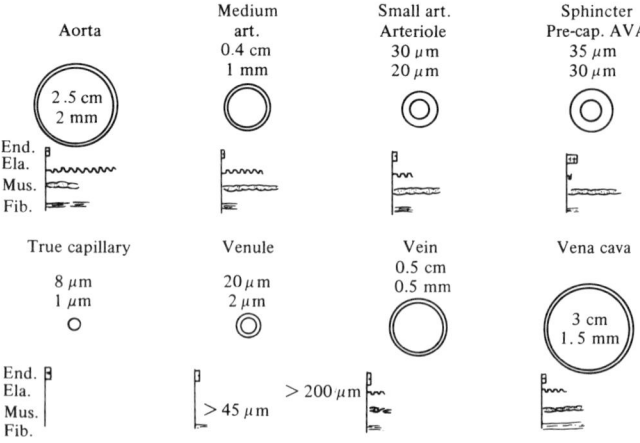

Fig. 54. Geometry and composition of blood vessel walls. (From Burton, 1972.)

6.1 Blood vessel walls

The motion of the vessel wall is restrained in all directions, especially in the longitudinal direction, due to vascular tethering. Thus, the effect of tethering should be taken into account in the rheology of blood vessels. Strictly speaking, blood vessels are not Hookean. Any component of stress plotted against any component of strain is a straight line for a Hookean material. Figure 55 shows the load–length curve of a circumferential strip of dog's aorta; it is clearly not a straight line; it is not even a single curve. Hence the blood vessel is not Hookean; it is not elastic but viscoelastic. However, the blood vessel would obey Hooke's law if we limited ourselves to a very small range of variation of stress and strain.

Cox (1979) pointed out that passive elements in blood vessels serve several very important roles. His results also indicate that the mechanical properties of blood vessels under conditions of active and passive smooth muscle are dependent upon a number of different quantities. The passive mechanical properties of blood vessels are determined by the relative connective tissue content, the fraction of collagen fibers supporting wall load, the mechanical

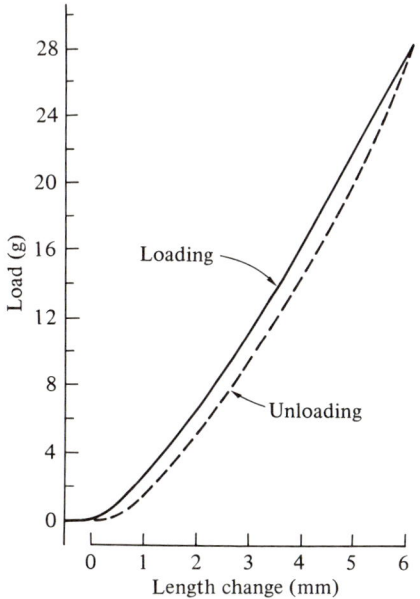

Fig. 55. Load–length curve of a circumferential strip. (From Tanaka & Fung, 1974.)

properties of the elastin and collagen matrices, and the arrangement and/or distribution of these connective tissue elements. Connective tissue elements also appear to contribute to the active stiffness of blood vessels, and collagen at least is involved in the intracellular transduction of cellular force development in vascular smooth muscle.

6.2 Forces in blood vessel walls

(a) Axial force and circumferential force

Let us take a segment of blood vessel of unit length bounded by two cross-sections, and consider the forces acting on the segment (Fig. 56). The force T_L acting on the cross-section is the axial force, and the total force T_c acting perpendicularly to the plane $ABB'A'$ is the circumferential force, usually called the *circumferential tension*. This can be regarded as a force acting per unit length BB' parallel to the axis. Thus, the dimensions of T_c are given by [force] [length]$^{-1}$, as with surface tension; the CGS unit of T_c is dyn cm^{-1}. The circumferential tension is assumed to be positive if it stretches in the circumferential direction, and negative if it is being compressed.

(b) Elastic tension and active tension

The circumferential tension in a blood vessel *in vivo* is, in general, composed of two different kinds of forces: (i) the elastic tension T_e due to passive deformation of the wall; (ii) the active

Fig. 56. Definition of a circumferential tension T_c and an axial force. T_L.

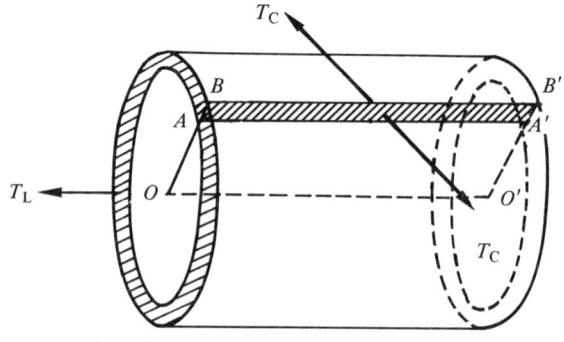

tension T_a due to the contraction of smooth muscle in the wall. The elastic tension can be positive or negative, but the active tension is always positive. The elastic tension is, of course, a function of the deformation of the wall.

6.3 General theory of circumferential tension

(a) *General formula*

Let us consider a straight cylindrical tube of uniform cross-section. Its inner and outer radius are r_1 and r_2 in the undeformed state. When the cylindrical tube is subjected to an internal pressure p_1 and an external pressure p_2, the corresponding inner and outer radii are r'_1 and r'_2, respectively. Here the shape of the circular cylinder is assumed to be maintained during the deformation. Our assumption is valid for a homogeneous wall of a blood vessel. Even for a wall that is not homogeneous, the assumption may be permitted provided the wall has an axial symmetry and uniformity.

For the balance of force in the cylindrical tube, it is convenient to consider a segment of tube bounded by two cross-sections and divided in half by a plane passing through the axis. In the upper half the resultant forces acting on the outer and inner surface of the cylinder are given by $2r'_2 p_2$ and $2r'_1 p_1$, respectively (Fig. 57). Then, for the equilibrium of the portion we have the relation:

Fig. 57. Equilibrium of a half portion of a blood vessel.

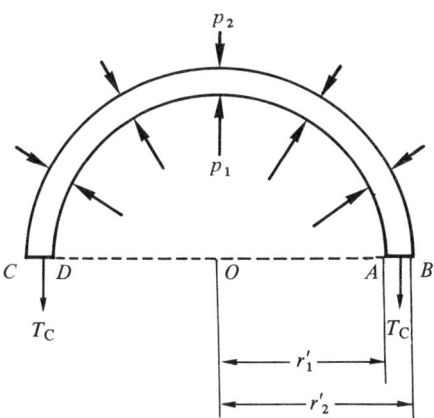

$$2r'_2 p_2 + 2T_c = 2r'_1 p_1$$

or

$$T_c = p_1 r'_1 - p_2 r'_2 \tag{6.1}$$

The above equation holds quite generally; it is valid irrespective of whether or not the wall is homogeneous, whether the wall is isotropic or anisotropic, and whether or not the wall is Hookean. This relation is often called *Oka–Azuma equation* (Oka, 1967; Oka & Azuma, 1970). It was also derived independently by Fung (1968).

Equation (6.1) can be rewritten as

$$T_c = (p_1 - p_2)r'_2 - p_1 r'_2 d \tag{6.2}$$

where d is the thickness ratio, defined by:

$$d = (r'_2 - r'_1)/r'_2 \tag{6.3}$$

(b) *Two limiting cases*
(i) Infinitely thin wall ($d = 0$).

The second term on the right-hand side of Eq. (6.2) vanishes. Then we have

$$T_c = (p_1 - p_2)r \tag{6.4}$$

where r stands for $r'_1 = r'_2$. Equation (6.4) is nothing other than Laplace's law. Burton (1951) used this equation in calculating the circumferential tension in a blood vessel wall from the transmural pressure $(p_1 - p_2)$ and the radius of the vessel, r. It must be emphasized that Laplace's law is valid only for blood vessels with infinitely thin walls, and always gives a positive value for the circumferential tension.

(ii) The internal pressure is equal to the external pressure ($p_1 = p_2$).

The first term of the right-hand side of Eq. (6.2) vanishes, and then we have

$$T_c = -p_1 r'_2 d$$

It is interesting to note that T_c is always negative in this case. The negative value of T_c indicates that the overall effect is a compression of the blood vessel. This is because the outer surface area of the wall is larger than the inner one.

6.3 General theory of circumferential tension

(c) *Relationship between Oka–Azuma equation and Laplace's law*

The Oka–Azuma equation (6.1) can be rewritten, except for the zero transmural pressure ($p_1 = p_2$), as follows:

$$T_c = m(p_1 - p_2)r'_2 \tag{6.5}$$

with the abbreviations:

$$m = 1 - (k/(k-1))d \tag{6.6}$$

$$k = p_1/p_2 \tag{6.7}$$

In the above, k is called the *pressure ratio*; it is always larger than unity. The quantity m is a dimensionless factor related to the deviation from Laplace's law in the circumferential tension. The above equation indicates that Laplace's law may provide a good approximation to the Oka–Azuma equation if and only if the non-dimensional parameter m is nearly equal to unity.

Figure 58 shows the plot m against d for a given value of k. It should be noted that m is positive or negative depending on whether d is less or greater than $1 - (1/k)$. The negative value of m means that the blood vessel is actually in a state of compression as a whole.

Table 3 gives a comparison of circumferential tensions calculated

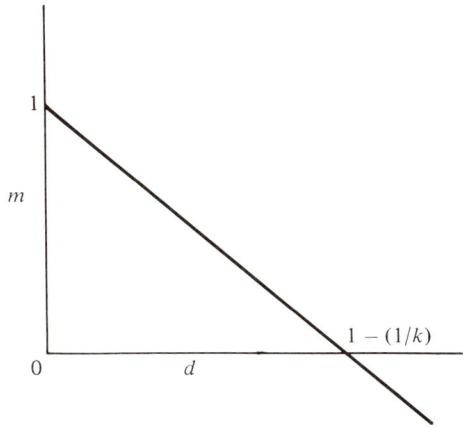

Fig. 58. The coefficient m vs. the thickness ratio d for a given pressure ratio k. (From Oka & Azuma, 1970.)

Table 3. *Circumferential tension calculated from Laplace's law and that from Oka–Azuma equation (From Azuma & Oka, 1971.)*

Blood vessel	Mean transmural pressure Δp(mm Hg)	Radius r, r'_1 (μm)	$T_c = \Delta p r$, (dyn cm^{-1})	Wall thickness (μm)	m	$T_c = p_1 r'_1 - p_2 r'_2$ (dyn cm^{-1})	τ 10^5(dyn cm^{-1})
Aorta and large arteries	100	1.3×10^4	1.7×10^5	1.3×10^3	$+0.22$	4.09×10^4	$+3.15$
Small distributing arteries	90	0.5×10^4	6.0×10^4	1×10^3	-0.57	-4.10×10^4	-4.10
Arterioles	60	0.15×10^4	1.2×10^3	50	-2.43	-3.89×10^3	-7.78
				30	-1.28	-1.84×10^3	-6.13
				15	-0.25	-330	-2.20
Capillaries	30	4	16	1.0	-4.26	-85.2	-8.52
				0.5	-1.92	-34.6	-6.92
				0.2	-0.25	-4.2	-2.10
Venules	20	10	26	1.0	-2.55	-72.9	-7.29
				0.4	-0.50	-13.5	-3.38
Veins	15	200	4.0×10^2	10	-1.46	-6.13×10^2	-6.13
				4	-0.01	-4.1	-0.10
Vena cava	10	1.6×10^4	2.1×10^4	0.2×10^3	$+0.05$	1.05×10^3	$+0.53$

6.3 General theory of circumferential tension

by Laplace's law with those calculated by the general equation (6.1). The first four items were transcribed from Burton's paper. In the table, it is assumed that the external pressure equals the atmospheric pressure, and the mean stress τ is calculated from

$$\tau = T_c/(r'_2 - r'_1) \tag{6.8}$$

As shown in the table, the signs of m are only positive in the largest arteries and vena cava. But the values are small, i.e. 0.22 in the former and only 0.05 in the latter. Thus, it is clear that Laplace's law greatly overestimates wall tension in these blood vessels. In other categories of blood vessel, the signs of m and, accordingly, the signs of tension, are all negative.

(d) Effect of pulsatile pressure

The general formula (6.1) was derived under the assumption that the wall is in static equilibrium. Actually, arteries are subjected to internal pressure which varies periodically. Let us estimate the effect of the motion of the wall. The motion of the upper half portion of the tube is described by the equation of motion:

$$M\ddot{y}_G = 2p_1 r'_1 - 2p_2 r'_2 - 2T_c \tag{6.9}$$

where M is the mass, and y_G is the distance of the center of gravity G from the axis of the tube.* The quantities M and y_G are given by

$$M = \frac{\pi}{2}\rho(r'^2_2 - r'^2_1) \tag{6.10}$$

$$y_G = \frac{2}{3}\frac{\rho}{M}(r'^3_2 - r'^3_1) \tag{6.11}$$

The radii r'_1, r'_2 may change periodically corresponding to changes in p_1. The external pressure p_2 is supposed to be kept nearly constant. Thus, if we denote the time average over one period by the bar, we can obtain the following result from Eq. (6.9):

$$\overline{T}_c = \overline{p_1 r'_1} - \overline{p_2 r'_2} \tag{6.12}$$

In the above, use has been made of the relations:

$$\overline{M\ddot{y}_G} = 0 \quad \overline{p_1 r'_1} \approx \bar{p}_1 \bar{r}'_1$$

---

*$\ddot{y}_G \equiv d^2 y_G/dt^2$

under the assumption that the amplitude of the oscillatory terms in p_1 and r'_1 are small in comparison with the mean values of p_1 and r_1. Therefore, we come to the conclusion that the general formula (6.1) is valid for the tube wall subjected to oscillatory internal pressure, provided that all the quantities in Eq. (6.1) are replaced by the quantities averaged over one period.

6.4 Stress distribution in blood vessel walls

Let us consider the stress distribution in a blood vessel wall in the cylindrical coordinate system (r, θ, z), where the z-axis coincides with the axis of the blood vessel. Let us denote the normal stress components by $\tau_r, \tau_\theta, \tau_z$ in the r-, θ-, z-directions, respectively.

The circumferential tension T_c is obtained by integrating the circumferential stress τ_θ over the thickness of the wall, as follows:

$$T_c = \int_{r'_1}^{r'_2} \tau_\theta \, dr \tag{6.13}$$

In general, the circumferential stress τ_θ is composed of elastic stress τ_θ^e and the active stress τ_θ^a due to the contraction of muscle. Then, the circumferential tension T_c can be described in the form:

$$T_c = \int_{r'_1}^{r'_2} \tau_\theta^e \, dr + \int_{r'_1}^{r'_2} \tau_\theta^a \, dr \tag{6.14}$$

It is very difficult to determine how the stress is distributed in a blood vessel, because the vessel wall is a complicated structure. Here we are concerned with two simple models of blood vessel wall. The active tension is not taken into consideration.

(a) Homogeneous, isotropic, Hookean wall

Let us examine the stress distribution in a homogeneous, isotropic, Hookean wall of a cylindrical tube which is subjected to the internal pressure p_1 and the external pressure p_2. The tube may be deformed so that the inner and outer radii change from r_1 and r_2 in the unstrained state to r'_1 and r'_2, respectively. If the strain is infinitesimal, r'_1 and r'_2 can be regarded as equal to r_1 and r_2, respectively.

According to the classical theory of elasticity, the normal stresses

6.4 Stress distribution in blood vessel walls

are given by

$$\tau_r = \frac{p_1 r_1^2 - p_2 r_2^2}{r_2^2 - r_1^2} - \frac{(p_1 - p_2) r_1^2 r_2^2}{r_2^2 - r_1^2} \frac{1}{r^2}$$

$$\tau_\theta = \frac{p_1 r_1^2 - p_2 r_2^2}{r_2^2 - r_1^2} + \frac{(p_1 - p_2) r_1^2 r_2^2}{r_2^2 - r_1^2} \frac{1}{r^2} \qquad (6.15)$$

$$\tau_z = \frac{p_1 r_1^2 - p_2 r_2^2}{r_2^2 - r_1^2}$$

In the above, use has been made of the boundary condition at the end of tube as follows:

$$\int_{r_1}^{r_2} \tau_z r \, dr = \tfrac{1}{2}(p_1 r_1^2 - p_2 r_2^2) \qquad (6.16)$$

The tangential stresses vanish, i.e. $\tau_{r\theta} = \tau_{\theta z} = \tau_{zr} = 0$. It should be noted that neither Young's modulus nor Poisson's ratio appear in the stress formulas.

If we consider the special case where $p_1 = p_2 = p$, then we have $\tau_r = \tau_\theta = \tau_z = -p$, indicating a uniform compressive stress throughout the wall. This is because the external pressure acts on larger surface area than the internal pressure. The compressive stress vanishes only when $p = 0$.

From Eqs. (6.13) and (6.15) we obtain the circumferential tension:

$$T_c = \int_{r_1}^{r_2} \tau_\theta \, dr = p_1 r_1 - p_2 r_2$$

This result is expected from Eq. (6.1), which is a general relationship valid of course for the present case.

Let us look at the relation between τ_θ and r. Since p_1 is greater than p_2, the second term on the right-hand side of Eq. (6.15) is always positive and decreases with the increase in r, while the first term of τ_θ is constant and may take a positive or negative value depending upon the values of p_1, p_2, r_1, and r_2. Therefore, with regard to the stress distribution in the tube wall, three cases can be distinguished (Fig. 59).

Case (a) τ_θ is always positive throughout the tube wall. This condition corresponds to $\tau_\theta(r_2) > 0$, i.e.

$$p_1 r_1^2 - p_2 r_2^2 + (p_1 - p_2) r_1^2 > 0 \qquad (6.17)$$

Case (b) τ_θ is positive in the inner region, but is negative in the outer region of the tube. This condition corresponds to $\tau_\theta(r_1) > 0$ and $\tau_\theta(r_2) < 0$, i.e.

$$p_1 r_1^2 - p_2 r_2^2 + (p_1 - p_2)r_2^2 > 0 \\ p_1 r_1^2 - p_2 r_2^2 + (p_1 - p_2)r_1^2 < 0 \quad (6.18)$$

Case (c) τ_θ is always negative throughout the tube wall. This condition corresponds to $\tau_\theta(r_1) < 0$, i.e.

$$p_1 r_1^2 - p_2 r_2^2 + (p_1 - p_2)r_2^2 < 0 \quad (6.19)$$

The above inequalities can be simplified by introducing dimensionless parameters:

$$k = p_1/p_2 \quad \text{and} \quad s = r_2/r_1 \quad (6.20)$$

k is the pressure ratio and s is the *radius ratio*, both being greater than unity. Then the inequality (6.17) is expressed as

$$k > \tfrac{1}{2}(1 + s^2) \quad (6.21)$$

Similarly, the inequalities (6.18) and (6.19) are expressed as

$$\frac{2s^2}{1+s^2} < k < \frac{1}{2}(1 + s^2) \quad (6.22)$$

$$k < \frac{2s^2}{1+s^2} \quad (6.23)$$

respectively.

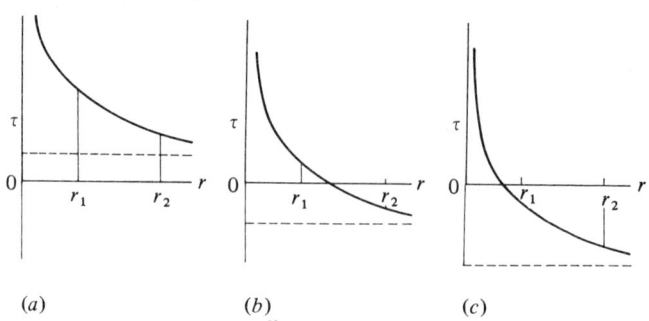

Fig. 59. Three cases of circumferential stress distribution in a Hookean tube wall. (From Oka & Azuma, 1970.)

6.4 Stress distribution in blood vessel walls

It is convenient to consider the sk-plane. The region $s > 1$, $k > 1$ on the sk-plane is now divided into three regions, A, B, and C by the two curves:

$$LM: \quad k = \tfrac{1}{2}(1 + s^2) \tag{6.24}$$

and

$$LN: \quad k = \frac{2s^2}{1 + s^2} \tag{6.25}$$

as in Fig. 60. The curves LM and LN are the graphs of Eqs. (6.24) and (6.25), respectively. Regions A, B and C correspond to the cases (a), (b) and (c). The curves LM and LN have a common tangent LT at the point $L(1, 1)$, i.e. $k = s$. The curve LN has an asymptote $k = 2$.

The stress distribution in a tube wall is shown schematically in Fig. 61.

Since Eq. (6.1) can be rewritten as

$$T_c = p_2 r'_1 (k - s) \tag{6.26}$$

the circumferential tension T_c vanishes on the tangent LT. The upper and lower regions of the tangent correspond to $T_c > 0$ and $T_c < 0$, respectively. Thus, the region B is divided by the tangent LT into two regions, B_1 and B_2. These correspond to case (b), but

Fig. 60. Sign of circumferential stress τ_θ in a Hookean wall on the sk-plane. (From Oka & Azuma, 1970.)

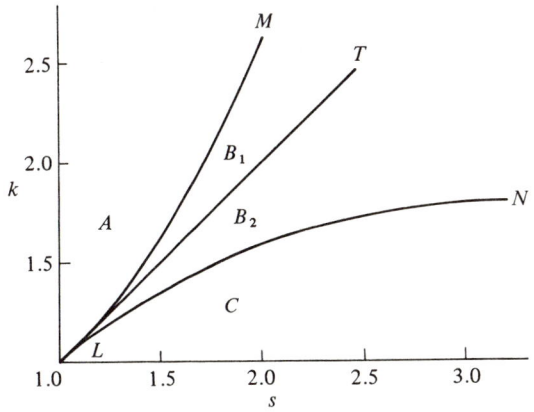

the circumferential tension is positive or negative in region B_1 or B_2, respectively. Hence we see that positive circumferential tension does not always mean that the stress is positive throughout the thickness of the wall. The same is true for negative circumferential tension. This can be predicted from Eq. (6.13).

(b) Wall with layered structures

Let us consider a tube which is composed of n homogeneous, isotropic, Hookean layers; let the ith layer be bounded by cylindrical surfaces of radius a_{i-1} and $a_i (> a_{i-1})$, $(i = 1, 2, \ldots, n)$; the inner and outer radii of the tube are $r_1 (= a_0)$ and $r_2 (= a_n)$, respectively. Let Young's modulus and Poisson's ratio of the ith layer be denoted by $E^{(i)}$ and $\sigma^{(i)}$, respectively. The tube wall is in equilibrium under the internal pressure p_1 and the external pressure p_2.

Then we can calculate the stress components $\tau_r^{(i)}$, $\tau_\theta^{(i)}$ and $\tau_z^{(i)}$ individually in the ith layer within the framework of the classical theory of elasticity as follows (Oka & Azuma, 1972):

$$\tau_r^{(i)} = \frac{E^{(i)}}{(1 + \sigma^{(i)})(1 - 2\sigma^{(i)})}\left[C_1^{(i)} + \sigma^{(i)} C - (1 - 2\sigma^{(i)})\frac{C_2^{(i)}}{r^2} \right]$$

$$\tau_\theta^{(i)} = \frac{E^{(i)}}{(1 + \sigma^{(i)})(1 - 2\sigma^{(i)})}\left[C_1^{(i)} + \sigma^{(i)} C + (1 - 2\sigma^{(i)})\frac{C_2^{(i)}}{r^2} \right]$$

$$\tau_z^{(i)} = \frac{E^{(i)}}{(1 + \sigma^{(i)})(1 - 2\sigma^{(i)})}[2\sigma^{(i)} C_1^{(i)} + (1 - 2\sigma^{(i)})C] \quad (6.27)$$

where $C_1^{(i)}$, $C_2^{(i)}$ and C are constants to be determined from the

Fig. 61. Three cases of circumferential stress distribution in a Hookean tube wall. (From Oka & Azuma, 1970.)

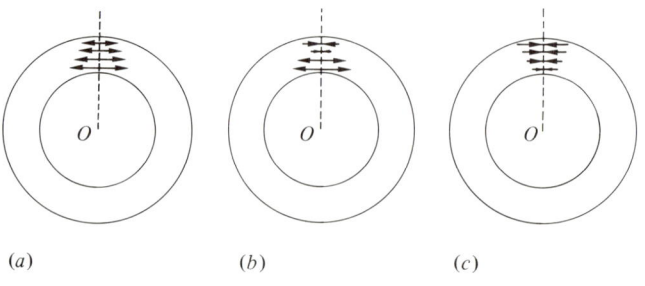

(a) (b) (c)

boundary conditions. The boundary conditions are: (i) the normal stress must be continuous at the boundaries, $r = a_i$, $r = r_1$, $r = r_2$; (ii) the circumferential component of strain must be continuous at the boundaries $r = a_i$; (iii) the axial force applied at the end of the tube is given. Here we do not determine the unknown constants, but consider only the circumferential tension T_c given by

$$T_c = \sum_{i=1}^{n} \int_{a_{i-1}}^{a_i} \tau_\theta^{(i)} dr \tag{6.28}$$

After some calculation, we have the final result:

$$T_c = p_1 r_1 - p_2 r_2$$

The above relation is nothing other than the Oka–Azuma equation (6.1). Thus, the Oka–Azuma equation is valid for cylindrical tubes of multilayered structures.

6.5 Incremental theory of blood vessel walls

As mentioned in Sect. 1, blood vessels are not Hookean. But if we consider a small increase in the stress and strain at a given state of deformation, the incremental strain is proportional to the incremental stress. Let us consider the *incremental theory* of blood vessels. Consider a segment of a cylindrical blood vessel with the middle radius R, length L, and wall thickness h, which is subjected to the internal and external pressures as well as the axial (symmetric) forces at both ends. The middle radius is the mean of the inner and outer radii. If the ratio R/h is 10 or larger, the blood vessel is regarded as thin-walled. We are here concerned with thin-walled blood vessels. It is convenient to consider the stress and strain in cylindrical coordinates (r, θ, z), where the z-axis coincides with the axis of the cylinder. If the wall is homogeneous and the end-effects are neglected, all the tangential stresses vanish. Accordingly, all the normal stresses become uniform along the θ- and z-directions, but vary along the r-direction.

(a) Incremental strain and stress

Let us denote the normal stress and strain components in the radial, circumferential, and axial directions in a particular state of the blood vessel by $\tau_r, \tau_\theta, \tau_z$, and $\gamma_r, \gamma_\theta, \gamma_z$, respectively.

The strain components at the middle surface of the wall are described by

$$\gamma_r = (h - h_0)/h_0 \qquad \gamma_\theta = (R - R_0)/R_0$$
$$\gamma_z = (L - L_0)/L_0 \qquad (6.29)$$

where R_0, L_0, and h_0 are the middle radius, length, and wall thickness in the natural (unstrained) state. Now, let us consider small increments in the normal stresses and strains in a given state and denote the *incremental stresses* and the *incremental strains* by P_r, P_θ, P_z, and e_r, e_θ, e_z in the radial, circumferential, and axial directions, respectively. If we denote the incremental value by Δ, the incremental stresses and strains are described by

$$P_r = \Delta \tau_r \qquad e_r = \frac{\Delta h}{h}$$
$$P_\theta = \Delta \tau_\theta \qquad e_\theta = \frac{\Delta R}{R} \qquad (6.30)$$
$$P_z = \Delta \tau_z \qquad e_z = \frac{\Delta L}{L}$$

There is a relationship among the incremental strains e_r, e_θ, e_z. The volume of the blood vessel wall must be kept constant under the deformation, due to its incompressibility. Since the volume of blood vessel is $2\pi R L h$, we have the incremental version:

$$\frac{\Delta R}{R} + \frac{\Delta L}{L} + \frac{\Delta h}{h} = 0$$

Hence,
$$e_r + e_\theta + e_z = 0 \qquad (6.31)$$

or
$$e_r = -e_\theta - e_z$$

thus we can calculate e_r from e_θ and e_z.

(b) Dynamic incremental strain and stress

When the blood vessel is subjected to an internal pressure which varies periodically, the incremental stresses and strains also vary periodically. Let the increase in the transmural pressure changing sinusoidally with time be represented in the complex

6.5 Incremental theory of blood vessel walls

form:

$$\Delta p = p_m e^{i\omega t} \tag{6.32}$$

where Δp is the incremental transmural pressure, p_m is the amplitude, and ω is the angular frequency. In general, the incremental strains and stresses are not in phase with the incremental transmural pressure, due to the viscoelasticity of the wall. Accordingly, we can describe the increments ΔR, ΔL as follows:

$$\Delta R = |\Delta R| e^{i(\omega t + \phi)}$$
$$\Delta L = |\Delta L| e^{i(\omega t + \psi)} \tag{6.33}$$

where ϕ and ψ are the phase differences. The incremental strains are easily expressed by putting the above equations into Eq. (6.30).

(c) Constitutive equations

Within a small range, the stress–strain relationship is linear. The incremental strains e_r, e_θ, e_z are generally expressed by linear combination of the incremental stresses P_r, P_θ, P_z in the complex representation:

$$\begin{aligned} e_r &= C_{rr} P_r - C_{r\theta} P_\theta - C_{rz} P_z \\ e_\theta &= -C_{\theta r} P_r + C_{\theta\theta} P_\theta - C_{\theta z} P_z \\ e_z &= -C_{zr} P_r - C_{z\theta} P_\theta + C_{zz} P_z \end{aligned} \tag{6.34}$$

The coefficients C_{ij} are in general complex; the negative signs before them are used for convenience. The coefficients C_{ij} are not all independent. If the matrix C_{ij} is symmetric, only six are independent. Further, the condition of incompressibility of a blood vessel wall requires three other relations among the six coefficients corresponding to the three independent incremental stresses. Consequently, only three coefficients $C_{rr}, C_{\theta\theta}, C_{zz}$ are independent.

(d) Incremental Young's modulus and Poisson's ratio

In the incremental theory, we define the *incremental Young's modulus* E_r, E_θ, E_z in the radial, circumferential, and axial directions, respectively, as follows:

$$E_r = \frac{P_r}{e_r} \qquad E_\theta = \frac{P_\theta}{e_\theta} \qquad E_z = \frac{P_z}{e_z} \tag{6.35}$$

Moreover, we define the *incremental Poisson's ratio* $\sigma_{ij}(i,j=r,\theta,z)$ as follows:

$$\sigma_{ij} = -\frac{e_i}{e_j} \tag{6.36}$$

The incremental Young's modulus and Poisson's ratio are related to the coefficients C_{ij} by the constitutive equation. To see this, let us examine some special cases. If $P_r = P_z = 0, P_\theta \neq 0$, we have $e_\theta = C_{\theta\theta} P_\theta$ in Eq. (6.34). Hence we have $E_\theta = 1/C_{\theta\theta}$. Similarly, we have the following relations:

$$E_r = \frac{1}{C_{rr}} \quad E_\theta = \frac{1}{C_{\theta\theta}} \quad E_z = \frac{1}{C_{zz}} \tag{6.37}$$

Note that the incremental Young's moduli E_r, E_θ, E_z are in general complex, corresponding to the complex coefficients C_{ij}.

In another special case, where $P_r = P_z = 0, P_\theta \neq 0$, we have the relation $-e_z/e_\theta = C_{z\theta}/C_{\theta\theta}$. Thus, we have the following relations for the incremental Poisson's ratios:

$$\sigma_{z\theta} = \frac{C_{z\theta}}{C_{\theta\theta}} \quad \sigma_{rz} = \frac{C_{rz}}{C_{zz}} \quad \sigma_{\theta r} = \frac{C_{\theta r}}{C_{rr}}$$
$$\sigma_{\theta z} = \frac{C_{\theta z}}{C_{zz}} \quad \sigma_{zr} = \frac{C_{zr}}{C_{rr}} \quad \sigma_{r\theta} = \frac{C_{r\theta}}{C_{\theta\theta}} \tag{6.38}$$

Note that $\sigma_{ij} \neq \sigma_{ji}$. The incremental Poisson's ratios are also complex.

(e) Determination of incremental constitutive coefficients

The incremental constitutive coefficients developed above can be determined from *in vivo* and *in vitro* experiments. Patel, Janicki & Carew (1969) evaluated *in vivo* coefficients from experiments on the aorta of an anesthetized dog. Figure 62 shows the incremental Young's moduli against the strains. Note that the elastic moduli increase with increasing strain and that, in general, $E_z > E_\theta > E_r$ at physiological pressures, indicating anisotropic behavior of the vessel wall. They also showed that the values of the incremental Poisson's ratios always averaged 0.5 because of

6.6 Nonlinear theory of elastic deformation

Since blood vessels have nonlinear elastic properties, we here apply the nonlinear theory to the thin-walled blood vessel, using the same notation as in the previous section. Instead of mean strains, we define mean stretch ratios in the radial, circumferential, and axial directions as follows:

$$\lambda_\theta = \frac{R}{R_0} \qquad \lambda_z = \frac{L}{L_0} \qquad \lambda_r = \frac{h}{h_0} \qquad (6.39)$$

In the nonlinear theory, it is convenient to introduce the *Green–St. Venant strains* defined by:

$$\overline{\gamma_\theta} = \tfrac{1}{2}(\lambda_\theta^2 - 1) \qquad \overline{\gamma_z} = \tfrac{1}{2}(\lambda_z^2 - 1) \qquad \overline{\gamma_r} = \tfrac{1}{2}(\lambda_r^2 - 1) \qquad (6.40)$$

The Green–St. Venant strains $\overline{\gamma_\theta}, \overline{\gamma_z}, \overline{\gamma_r}$ vanish in the undeformed

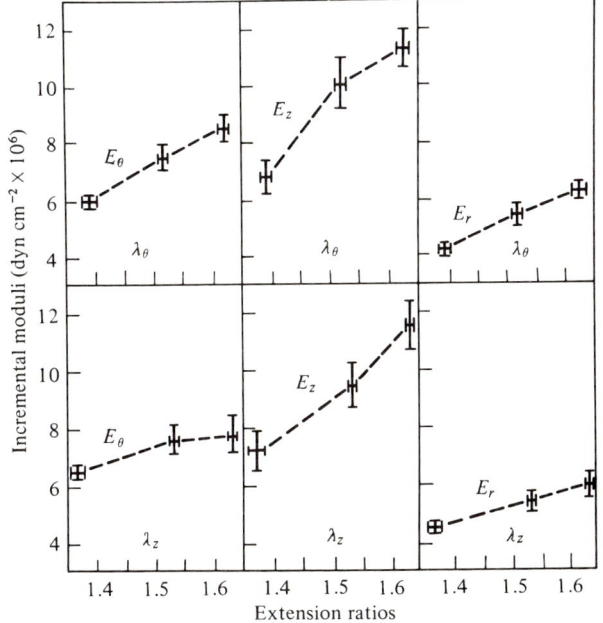

Fig. 62. Incremental Young's modulus vs. the stretch ratios. (From Patel *et al.*, 1969.)

state and are approximately equal to the conventional strains $\gamma_\theta, \gamma_z, \gamma_r$ when these are infinitesimal.

If the deformation process of a perfectly elastic material (without internal dissipation) is adiabatic, i.e. it does not exchange heat with its surroundings, then the excess of the mechanical work done over the increase in kinetic energy is stored in the body as strain energy. The strain energy per unit initial volume is a function of the state of deformation only, and is referred to as the *strain energy density function*. It is measured in dyn cm^{-2}, like stress.

Let us express the state of deformation of an elastic body by the Green–St. Venant strains, and for simplicity use the abbreviation:

$$a = \overline{\gamma_\theta} \qquad b = \overline{\gamma_z} \qquad c = \overline{\gamma_r} \tag{6.41}$$

Then the strain energy density function can be written as

$$W = W(a, b, c) \tag{6.42}$$

Now we are concerned, in particular, with an incompressible material for which W is a function only of λ_θ and λ_z, or a and b. It can then be shown that the stresses obtained are as follows:

$$\begin{aligned}\tau_\theta - \tau_r &= (1 + 2a)\frac{\partial W}{\partial a} \\ \tau_z - \tau_r &= (1 + 2b)\frac{\partial W}{\partial b}\end{aligned} \tag{6.43}$$

The functional form of W is a matter of primary concern. Vaishnav, Young, Janicki & Patel (1972) assumed that W can be approximated by a polynomial in a, b, and c. Now the condition of incompressibility is $\lambda_\theta \lambda_z \lambda_r = 1$, i.e.

$$(1 + 2a)(1 + 2b)(1 + 2c) = 1 \tag{6.44}$$

Thus, we can express c in terms of an infinite series in a and b. Finally, we get the following expression for W:

$$W = Aa^2 + Bab + Cb^2 + Da^3 + Ea^2b + Fab^2 + Gb^3 \tag{6.45}$$

where the fourth-degree terms are eliminated. The constant term corresponding to the constrained state can be set equal to zero. In addition, it can be shown that the first-order term can also be set equal to zero, provided that the undeformed state is stress-free. They performed experiments *in vitro* on specimens from four dogs to test the applicability of the nonlinear theory. For the 7-constant theory based on Eq. (6.45), the following average values were obtained for the material parameters:

$A = 0.412 \ (\pm 0.066)$ $B = -0.067 \ (\pm 0.131)$
$C = 0.191 \ (\pm 0.059)$ $D = -0.055 \ (\pm 0.036)$
$E = 0.162 \ (\pm 0.051)$ $F = 0.179 \ (\pm 0.103)$
$G = 0.099 \ (\pm 0.087)$

They experimentally tested the nonlinear 3-, 7-, and 12-constant theories, and found that the *7-constant theory* appears to be satisfactory for most practical purposes.

Instead of a polynominal of the type in Eq. (6.45), Fung (Fung, Fronek & Patitucci, 1979) proposed an exponential function of the form:

$$W = \tfrac{1}{2} C \exp(\alpha a^2 + 2\beta ab + \gamma b^2) \qquad (6.46)$$

where C, α, β, γ are material constants.

6.7 Tethering effect on the stresses in blood vessels

The axial tethering of the blood vessel has a marked influence on the stress distribution in its wall. Let us consider a theory of the tethering effect (Chu & Oka, 1973). We assume that the blood vessel is a hollow cylindrical tube in equilibrium under constant internal and external pressure; its shape is maintained under deformation along with the additional constraint that it has a constant longitudinal stretch, k.

In order to consider large deformation, we regard the blood vessel wall as a neo-Hookean material. For simplicity, we further assume that the wall is homogeneous, isotropic and incompressible.

Consider a cylindrical tube which in the undeformed state has length L, inner radius A, and outer radius B (Fig. 63). Next consider the hollow cylindrical tube deformed under constant internal pressure p_1 and external pressure p_2, and let the corresponding inner and outer radii of the tube be denoted by a and b, respectively.

The principal stretch ratios λ_1, λ_2 and λ_3 in the radial, circumferential and axial directions, respectively, are

$$\lambda_1 = \frac{dr}{dR} \qquad \lambda = \lambda_2 = \frac{r}{R} \qquad \lambda_3 = \frac{z}{Z} = k \qquad (6.47)$$

The condition of incompressibility requires that

$$\lambda_1 \lambda_2 \lambda_3 = 1$$

or

$$kr\, dr = R\, dR$$

Integration gives

$$kr^2 = R^2 + D \qquad (6.48)$$

where D is a constant.

The strain energy density function W for a *neo-Hookean material* is

$$W = \tfrac{1}{2} G (I_1 - 3) \qquad (6.49)$$

where G is the initial shear modulus, and I_1 is the strain invariant:

$$I_1 = \lambda_1^2 + \lambda_2^2 + \lambda_3^2 \qquad (6.50)$$

The stress distribution in the tube wall is calculated as follows:

$$\begin{aligned}
\tau_\theta &= G\left[\lambda^2 - \frac{1}{k} \ln \lambda - \frac{1}{2k^2 \lambda^2} + \frac{\text{const}}{G} \right] \\
\tau_z &= G\left[k^2 - \frac{1}{k} \ln \lambda - \frac{1}{2k^2 \lambda^2} + \frac{\text{const}}{G} \right] \\
\tau_r &= G\left[\frac{1}{2k^2 \lambda^2} - \frac{1}{k} \ln \lambda + \frac{\text{const}}{G} \right]
\end{aligned} \qquad (6.51)$$

Fig. 63. Stress and deformation in a neo-Hookean tube. (From Chu & Oka, 1973.)

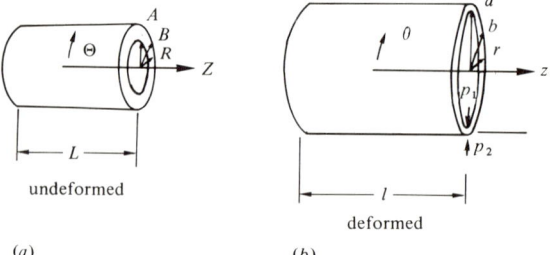

(a) undeformed

(b) deformed

6.7 Tethering effect on stresses in blood vessels

The boundary conditions are:

$$r = a: \quad \tau_r = -p_1$$
$$r = b: \quad \tau_r = -p_2 \tag{6.52}$$

The unknown constants D and const/G can be determined using Eqs. (6.51) and (6.52). The circumferential tension, T_c, can then be obtained by integrating τ_θ across the thickness of the wall, i.e.

$$\begin{aligned} T_c &= \int_a^b \tau_\theta \, dr \\ &= G \int_a^b \left\{ \frac{r^2/k}{r^2 - D/k} - \frac{1}{k} \ln\left[\frac{r}{(kr^2 - D)^{1/2}}\right] \right. \\ &\quad \left. - \frac{r^2 - D/k}{2kr^2} + \frac{\text{const}}{G} \right\} dr \end{aligned} \tag{6.53}$$

After integrating and substituting the values of D and const/G, we get exactly the result:

$$T_c = p_1 a - p_2 b \tag{6.54}$$

which conforms with the general formula (6.1). Equation (6.54) shows $T_c \gtrless 0$ depending on whether $p_1/p_2 \gtrless b/a$.

It is interesting to compare the strain energy density function for a neo-Hookean material with its approximation by a polynomial in a and b. I_1 is given by

$$\begin{aligned} I_1 &= \lambda_\theta^2 + \lambda_z^2 + \lambda_r^2 \\ &= (1 + 2a) + (1 + 2b) + (1 + 2a)^{-1}(1 + 2b)^{-1} \end{aligned}$$

On expanding the expression $(1 + 2a)^{-1}(1 + 2b)^{-1}$ in terms of powers of a and b, and neglecting small quantities, namely the third and higher degree terms, we get

$$I_1 = 3 + 4(a^2 + ab + b^2)$$

or

$$W = 2G(a^2 + ab + b^2) \tag{6.55}$$

This expression corresponds to the 3-constant theory with $A = B = C = 2G$. The equality $A = B = C$ corresponds to the isotropic property of the neo-Hookean material.

6.8 Some rheological models of blood vessels

(a) *Vascular nonlinearity*

A number of experimental studies have been done to describe the rheological properties of blood vessels. These include in-vitro and in-vivo studies of length–tension relationships on vascular strips cut at an angle to the axis of blood vessels, or of pressure–diameter relationships on intact segments of blood vessels. There is much experimental evidence of vascular nonlinearity in the length–tension relationship and the pressure–diameter relationship. Most of these relationships apply to blood vessels when the smooth muscle is passive; a different response may occur when the smooth muscle is activated.

Two kinds of empirical law have been used to describe nonlinear behavior in the length–tension and the pressure–diameter relationships: a nonlinear power law, and an exponential law. The exponential law seems preferable because it is theoretically simpler (Fung et al. 1979).

Okumura et al. (1976) introduced a logarithmic equation in the pressure–diameter relationship in order to determine the effect of smooth muscle on the mechanical properties of arteries, as follows:

$$\ln(p/p_s) = \beta(D/D_s - 1) \tag{6.56}$$

where p_s is the standard pressure and D_s is the outer diameter of the artery at the standard pressure (which is taken as 100 mm Hg). The quantity β is a dimensionless parameter which is a measure of the *stiffness* of the wall. Hayashi et al. (1980a) compared the stiffness of human intracranial arteries and their age-related variation with those of extracranial arteries using the above relation.

Niimi et al. (1975) proposed a nonlinear model to describe the pressure–diameter relationship of blood vessels at a given state as follows:

$$\Delta R = C_1 \Delta p + C_2(\Delta p^2 - \overline{\Delta p^2}) \tag{6.57}$$

where Δp and ΔR are the increments in the transmural pressure p and the middle radius R; C_1 and C_2 are constants, and the bar over Δp^2 represents the time average.

6.8 Some rheological models of blood vessels

(b) *Vascular viscoelasticity*

Blood vessels generally exhibit viscoelastic properties, or time-dependent phenomena. Viscoelastic properties of blood vessels have been studied in two ways: transient responses in the time domain to changes in length (diameter) or changes in force (pressure), and responses to sinusoidal variation in length (diameter) in the frequency domain. Mathematically, studies in the time and frequency domains are transformable. Thus, studies in the frequency domain seem preferable because they are simpler and less subject to experimental errors (Cox, 1979).

Generally, in response to a step increase in force, the length of a blood vessel wall will immediately increase. If the force is held constant, the length of the blood vessel wall slowly increases to a larger value. Plotting the change of length against time under such

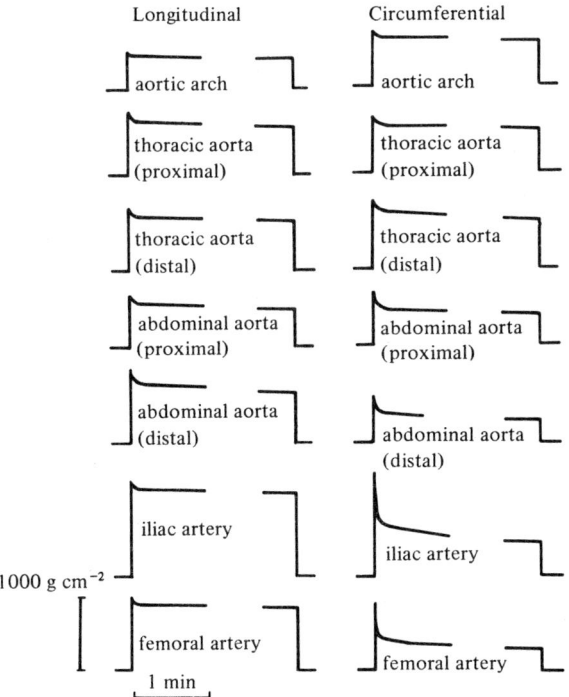

Fig. 64. Stress relaxation in different arteries. (From Azuma & Hasegawa, 1971.)

circumstances produces a function that is nearly exponential. The secondary decrease in force following a step increase in length is called *stress relaxation*. On the other hand, the secondary increase in length is called *creep*. These are two manifestations of viscoelastic properties of blood vessels.

The degree of viscoelasticity is evaluated by the magnitude of the stress relaxation following a step increase in length. Azuma & Hasegawa (1971) carried out the stress relaxation test on longitudinal and circumferential strips. Figure 64 shows the variation of the stress relaxation in different arteries. In the relaxation pattern, considerable differences are observed in the arterial system. The stress relaxation in the circumferential direction is always much larger than the stress relaxation in the longitudinal direction. Also, the degree of stress relaxation increases progressively from the ascending aorta down to the femoral artery. A close relationship may exit between the amount of muscle present in a given blood vessel and the degree of stress relaxation.

Figure 65 shows schematically an attempt to relate the observed mechanical properties to morphological structures. It was worked out on the basis of rheological and histological results. The more peripheral the portion, the more the number of turns in the smooth

Fig. 65. Diagram for structures of different arteries. (From Azuma & Hasegawa, 1971.)

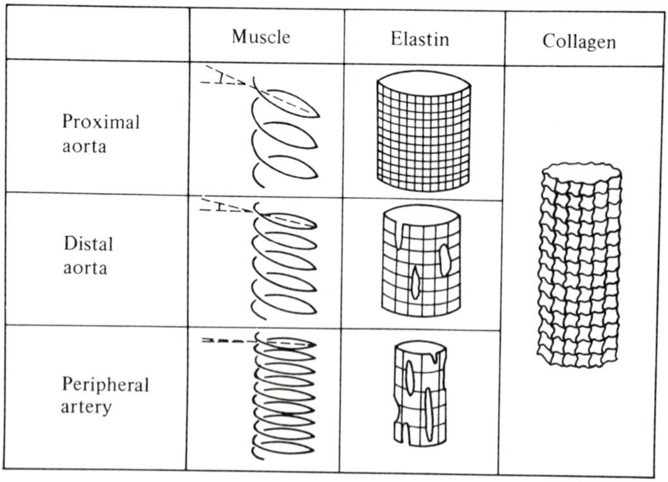

	Muscle	Elastin	Collagen
Proximal aorta			
Distal aorta			
Peripheral artery			

6.8 Some rheological models of blood vessels

muscle helix and the less the value of angle θ. The net work structure of elastin fibers becomes sparser in the more peripheral portions, with an increasing number of longitudinal cracks. Collagen fibers which form a network structure are in a crimped state, so that they can be stressed only after an overstretching which is sufficient to straighten all crimps.

A number of attempts have been made to describe viscoelastic behavior including stress relaxation in terms of rheological models. Three rheological models have been used for this purpose: the Maxwell model, the Kelvin model, and the three-element model. However, creep and stress relaxation curves recorded experimentally do not seem to follow the predictions. This is probably due to oversimplification; further, some elements are required to represent the true viscoelastic nature of blood vessels.

(c) Pseudoelasticity

In general, blood vessels are capable of large deformation, and show nonlinear elasticity. Moreover, they are not elastic in the strict sense of the word, but inelastic. The stress–strain curves differ for loading and unloading, which correspond to increasing load and decreasing load, respectively. In practice, however, the stress–strain relationships are rather insensitive to the strain rate. This also seems to be a general feature of other soft tissues.

Hysteresis is closely related to viscoelasticity, and the area of the hysteresis loop indicates the loss of mechanical energy during one cycle. Thus, strictly speaking, the strain energy density function is not applicable to blood vessels. However, we may treat the blood vessel as one elastic material in loading and another elastic material in unloading. Thus, we may use the theory of elasticity to consider an inelastic material. To remind us that we are really dealing with an inelastic material, we call it *pseudoelasticity*, after Fung *et al.* (1979)

7

Pulsatile flow

7.1 Pulse

The blood flow in blood vessels has so far been regarded as a steady flow. In fact, the blood flow in microvessels can be treated approximately as a steady flow, where the pressure gradient becomes constant with respect to time. In the aorta and large arteries, however, the blood pressure at a given site varies periodically, with the period corresponding to the heart beat.

The heart acts as a pump whose elastic, muscular walls contract rhythmically and thereby force blood through the vascular system. Blood flow is pulsatile due to the periodic action of the heart, which beats about 70 times a minute in a man at rest. As a result of ventricular contraction, a pressure pulse passes through the vascular system. Figure 66 shows the main features of the aortic pressure in man. Between points C and A the left ventricle is contracting and pushing about 60 ml of blood into the aorta. The pressure in the aorta rises rapidly to its maximum value of about 120 mm Hg. As the left heart relaxes, the pressure in the left ventricle falls below the aortic pressure, causing the valve between the left ventricle and the aorta to close at point B. Between points B and C the left heart relaxes and the aortic pressure falls to its minimum point C, around 80 mm Hg. The pressure at A is called the *systolic pressure*, p_s, and the pressure at C the *diastolic pressure*, p_d.

The difference between systolic and diastolic pressures, Δp ($\Delta p = p_s - p_d$), is called the *pulse pressure*. The time average, $\bar{p}$, of the blood pressure is the mean pressure, which is not equal to the arithmetical mean, $\frac{1}{2}(p_s + p_d)$, because the pressure does not form a sinusoidal wave. The nature of the pressure pulse in various parts of the vascular system is an important diagnostic tool in cardiovascular diseases.

Cardiac output is usually defined as the volume of blood pumped by the heart each minute. *Heart rate* is the number of heart beats per minute. *Stroke volume* is the volume of blood ejected by a ventricle. Thus, cardiac output is the product of stroke volume and heart rate.

7.2   Theoretical studies of pulse waves

The propagation of pulse waves nas long been studied theoretically by many investigators. This brief and general survey is made from several viewpoints.

(*a*) *Fluid*

It is simplest to treat blood as an inviscid fluid; this way was chosen by all investigators in the nineteenth century, including Young (1808). In the twentieth century, the viscous effects of blood were taken into account by Witzig (1914) and most investigators.

It was found by Scott Blair in 1959 that blood obeys Casson's equation. In recent years, experimental evidence has been accumulated to show that blood exhibits viscoelastic behavior. This non-Newtonian behavior of blood is important for blood flow in microvessels, where the flow velocity becomes extremely small. Yet the blood in pulsatile flow through large arteries may be regarded as a Newtonian fluid.

(*b*) *Shape of blood vessels*

Blood vessels have an extremely complex geometry. They

Fig. 66. Aortic pressure change in man. (From the National Cardiovascular Center Hospital, Japan.)

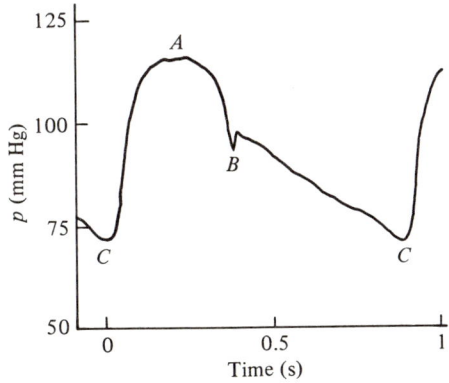

are branched and curved, and their size varies along the vascular tree. It is difficult to treat the whole blood vessel system theoretically. Thus, it is customary to choose a straight, unbranched, circular cylindrical tube of uniform thickness as a theoretical model of a blood vessel.

Blood flow in curved and/or branched vessels may differ, of course, from that in a straight one. Effects of curvature and branching may be neglected in the sites, especially microvessels, where the influence of the centrifugal force becomes negligible.

(c) Rheological properties of blood vessel walls

In order to treat the propagation of pressure waves theoretically, the blood vessel wall cannot be regarded as rigid, because the wave velocity would then become infinite. Thus, the artery wall has been treated as an elastic body since Young.

It is simplest, of course, to consider the wall as having Hookean elasticity. In the aorta and large arteries, the walls show nonlinear elasticity. The wall may then be treated, for simplicity, as having neo-Hookean elasticity. Going one step further, the viscoelasticity of the wall has been taken into account in the refined theory of pulse waves.

(d) Wall thickness

The wall thickness, h, of an artery is generally thin compared with its diameter. The arterioles are exceptions. In most theoretical studies, it has been assumed that the wall thickness is kept constant in the course of the wave propagation. When pulse waves propagate through the artery, the diameter varies with the periodic change of internal pressure. Then, the circumferential stretch due to the increase in diameter must cause a contraction in the radial direction under the condition of incompressibility of the wall. Therefore, the assumption that $h = $ const must be used with caution.

(e) Equation of motion

There are two ways of writing the equation of motion. The first is the quasi-one-dimensional way, in which a portion of fluid bounded by two neighboring cross-sections is considered as a whole. This must be supplemented by the relationship between the radius of the artery and the transmural pressure at the portion, which is usually based on a straight uniform cylindrical tube. Theoretical studies in the early days, from Young onwards, were of this type.

Most theoretical studies in the twentieth century belong to another category, which consists of three steps. In the first step, one uses the Navier–Stokes equation and the equation of continuity of an incompressible fluid. Because of the mathematical difficulties, the Navier–Stokes equation is often linearized.

In the second step, one writes the equation of motion for the wall. The equation of motion includes the effects of the elastic force due to deformation and of the viscous force due to fluid flow. Lamb (1898) expressed the elastic force in the widely used form of a thin-walled tube subjected to small strains under the condition of constant thickness.

In the third step, one considers the boundary conditions at the inner surface of the tube. The no-slip condition is usually adopted.

(f) *Influence of tethering*

Since blood vessels are embedded in the tissues, the motion of the vessel wall is influenced by the constraints of the tissue. The tethering effect may be particularly marked for the axial motion of the wall.

7.3 Oscillatory flow in a rigid tube

Let a long rigid tube of uniform circular cross-section be filled with an incompressible Newtonian fluid. The flow of a fluid through a tube under the influence of a periodic pressure difference is called *oscillatory flow*.

We denote the coordinate in the direction of the axis of the tube by z, and the radial distance from it by r. Since the radial velocity vanishes, and the axial velocity u is independent of z, it follows from the Navier–Stokes equation that the pressure gradient $\partial p/\partial z$ depends neither on z nor r, but is a function of time t only.

We here assume that the pressure gradient is harmonic:

$$-\frac{\partial p}{\partial z} = A \cos \omega t \qquad (7.1)$$

where a denotes a constant. If we use complex notation:

$$-\frac{\partial p}{\partial z} = A\, e^{i\omega t} \tag{7.2}$$

then the axial velocity u is obtained under no-slip condition at the wall as follows:

$$u(r,t) = \frac{AR^2}{i^3\alpha^2\eta}\left[1 - \frac{J_0(\alpha i^{3/2} y)}{J_0(\alpha i^{3/2})}\right] e^{i\omega t} \tag{7.3}$$

Here J_0 denotes the Bessel function of the first kind and of zero order, R is the inner radius of the tube, y is the normalized radial distance r/R, α is a dimensionless quantity defined by

$$\alpha = R(\omega/\nu)^{1/2} \tag{7.4}$$

and ν is the kinematic viscosity η/ρ. Equation (7.3) was obtained by

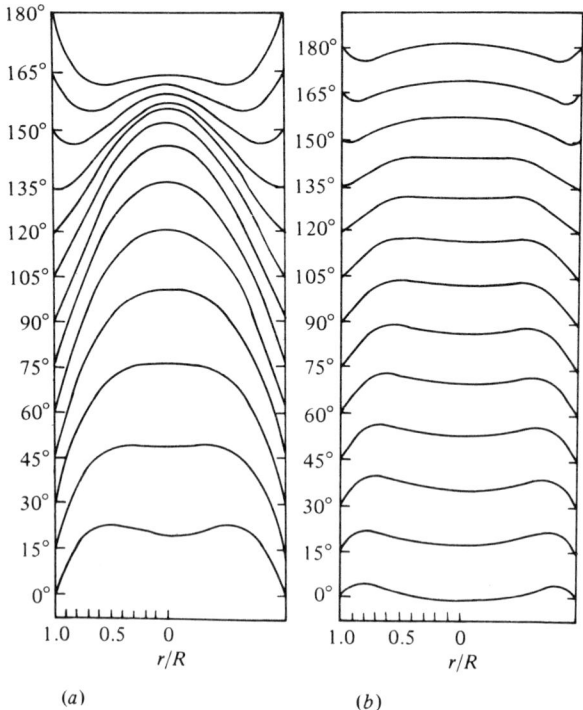

Fig. 67. Velocity profiles in an oscillatory flow in a rigid tube. (From Hale et al., 1955.)

(a) (b)

Womersley (1955), Uchida (1956), and others independently: α is usually called the *Womersley parameter*.

Womersley also integrated Eq. (7.3) to give the flow rate Q:

$$Q = \frac{\pi R^4}{\eta} \frac{A}{i^3 \alpha^2} \left[1 - \frac{2 J_1(\alpha i^{3/2})}{\alpha i^{3/2} J_0(\alpha i^{3/2})} \right] e^{i\omega t} \tag{7.5}$$

where J_1 is the Bessel function of the first kind and of the first order. He further computed $u(r, t)$ and Q by expressing the results in modulus and phase form.

Figure 67 shows the velocity profiles at intervals of 15° over a half cycle. The frequency in (b) is four times that in (a). Note that reversal of flow starts in the laminae near the wall. In (b) one can see the marked flattening of the profile in the central region of the tube, and the great reduction in amplitude.

The Womersley parameter, α, varies considerably along the arterial tree. In the aorta it is larger than 10, whilst in capillaries it is of the order of 10^{-3}.

7.4 Wave propagation in elastic tubes

(a) Wave velocity and attenuation

Many studies have been done of wave propagation in arteries. Here we introduce a linear theory of wave propagation in an infinitely long elastic tube, which was developed by Womersley.

Let us use the cylindrical coordinates (r, ϕ, z), where z coincides with the axis of the cylinder. Assuming axial symmetry, the fluid's axial velocity, u, and radial velocities, v, and the pressure, p, are determined by the linearized Navier–Stokes equation together with the equation of continuity. The axial displacement ρ and the radial displacement ξ of the wall are determined by the equation of motion for the wall. In addition, the no-slip condition is imposed at the wall. Womersley limited himself to periodic solutions $\exp(i\omega(t - z/c))$ for u, v, p, ρ and ξ, in which c is the *complex velocity* of wave propagation, and ω is the angular frequency. Insertion of the periodic solutions into the equations of motion and the equation of continuity, together with the boundary conditions, gave c^2 as follows:

$$\frac{Eh}{R\rho c^2} = G \pm [G^2 - (1 - \sigma^2)J]^{1/2} \tag{7.6}$$

where

$$G = \frac{\frac{5}{4} - \sigma}{1 - F} + \frac{k}{2} + \sigma - \frac{1}{4} \tag{7.7}$$

$$J = \frac{1 + 2k}{1 - F} - 1 \tag{7.8}$$

$$k = \frac{h}{R} \tag{7.9}$$

$$F = \frac{2J_1(\alpha i^{3/2})}{\alpha i^{3/2} J_0(\alpha i^{3/2})} \tag{7.10}$$

In the above equations E is Young's modulus and σ is Poisson's ratio for the wall. h is the constant wall thickness, and R is the inner radius of the tube in the undisturbed state. ρ is the density of blood and v is the kinematic viscosity of blood. Note that the density of the wall is assumed to be equal to that of the fluid.

Let us further denote

$$\frac{Eh}{2R\rho c^2} = X - iY \tag{7.11}$$

$$c_0 = \frac{Eh}{2\rho R} \tag{7.12}$$

Note that c_0, defined by Eq. (7.12), is usually known as the *Moens–Korteweg formula* for pulse wave velocity. This formula was derived by Young (1808), Weber (1866), and Resal (1876) for an incompressible inviscid fluid. Equation (7.11) can be written as

$$c_0/c = X - iY \tag{7.13}$$

Hence we have

$$\exp i\omega\left(t - \frac{z}{c}\right) = \exp\left(\frac{-2\pi Y}{X}\right)\frac{z}{\lambda} \exp i\omega\left(t - \frac{z}{c_1}\right)$$

where

$$c_1 = \frac{c_0}{X}, \quad \lambda = \frac{2\pi c}{\omega} \tag{7.14}$$

c_1 is the phase velocity, λ is the wavelength and $\exp(-2\pi Y/X)$ the

7.4 Wave propagation in elastic tubes

fraction to which the amplitude of a wave is reduced after travelling one wavelength. Both X and Y are functions of α, k, and σ. Womersley prepared tables of $1/X$, $2\pi Y/X$, and $\exp(-2\pi Y/X)$ as functions of α ranging from 1 to 10 for a number of values of k and σ. The phase velocity c_0 does not depend on the frequency, while the phase velocity c_1 depends on the frequency through the Womersley parameter α.

As α increases, the phase velocity c_1 approaches the phase velocity for an inviscid fluid. For a given tube and frequency, $\alpha \to \infty$ is equivalent to $\nu \to 0$. For a given tube and fluid, $\alpha \to \infty$ is equivalent to $\omega \to \infty$, and one can see that as the frequency increases, the inertial effect predominates over the viscous effect.

For a pulse wave whose waveform is not sinusoidal, the pressure wave at a given site can be expanded into Fourier series:

$$p = A_0 + \sum_{n=1}^{\infty} \left(A_n \cos \frac{2\pi nt}{T} + B_n \sin \frac{2\pi nt}{T} \right) \qquad (7.15)$$

Then each sinusoidal wave of different frequency propagates not only with different phase velocity but also with different attenuation constant. This indicates that the pulse wave changes in the waveform as it propagates.

Womersley studied the influence of tethering on the wave velocity and attenuation constant. He replaced, after Morgan & Ferranti (1955), the wall thickness h by $H(>h)$ to account for the inertial effect of the tissue in which the arteries are embedded. In order to express the axial constraint of the tethering of the artery, he introduced the concept of natural frequency $\omega/2\pi$. It can then be shown that k in Eq. (7.9) should be replaced by

$$K = \frac{h}{R} \frac{H}{h} \left(1 - \frac{\omega_0^2}{\omega^2} \right) \qquad (7.16)$$

which reduces to Eq. (7.9) if $H = h$ and $\omega_0 = 0$.

Figure 68 shows the variation of c_1/c_0 and $\exp(-2\pi Y/X)$ with α in an elastic tube, subject to varying degrees of constraint and filled with a viscous fluid. $K = 0$ represents a very thin unconstrained tube, $K = -\infty$ a tube with complete axial constraint, and $K = -2$ a tube with a small degree of constraint. In each curve, Poisson's ratio is taken as $\sigma = 0.5$. It should be noted that for $\alpha > 3$ the ratio

c_1/c_0 is close to unity in all three cases. For very small tubes, α is close to zero, and the wave attenuation becomes very marked.

Womersley further studied the effect of viscoelasticity of the wall, and found that both wave velocity and attenuation constant were increased by introducing the effect of the viscous properties of the wall. An intuitive explanation for the attenuation seems to be difficult.

(b) Peaking and steepening

McDonald (1974) illustrated the simultaneous change in amplitude and form of the pressure and flow waves at five sites from

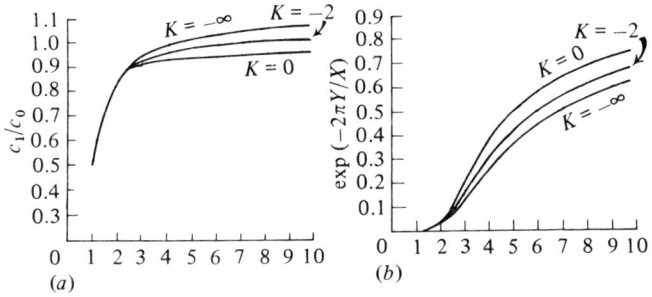

Fig. 68. Effect of tethering on wave velocity and attenuation in an elastic tube. (From Womersley, 1957.)

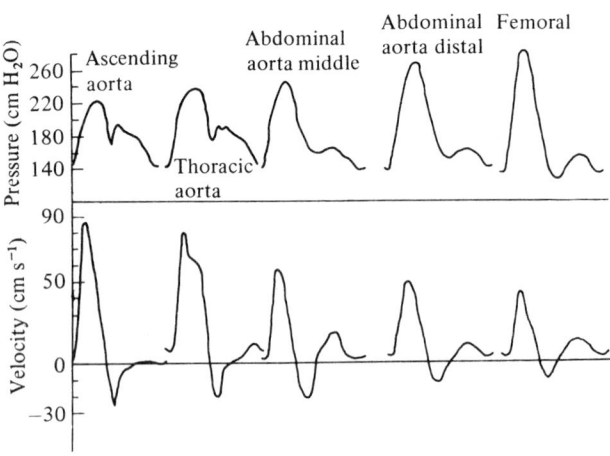

Fig. 69. Peaking and steepening of pressure waves and the progressive decrease of blood velocity. (From McDonald, 1974.)

the ascending aorta to the femoral artery (Fig. 69). As can be seen, the overall pressure oscillation increases as it travels away from the heart, which is known as *peaking*. The waveform becomes narrower as it travels away from the heart, which is known as *steepening*. These phenomena were formerly thought to be caused by the reflection of waves; but it is now believed that they are due to the nonlinearity in the Navier–Stokes equation.

It can be seen from Fig. 69 that the oscillation of flow velocity shows a progressive decrease. This is due to the increase in impedance with increasing distance from the heart.

7.5 Pressure–flow relationship

Let us examine the pressure–flow relationship in arteries using the same notation. For a forward wave of pressure:

$$p = A \exp[i\omega(t - z/c)] \tag{7.17}$$

the axial velocity u is obtained at an arbitrarily chosen point $z = 0$ as follows:

$$u = \frac{A}{\rho c}\left[1 + \chi \frac{J_0(i^{3/2} y\alpha)}{J_0(i^{3/2}\alpha)}\right] e^{i\omega t} \tag{7.18}$$

where

$$\chi = \frac{c^2(1 - \sigma^2)}{c_0^2(F - 2\sigma)} - \frac{1 - 2\sigma}{F - 2\sigma} \tag{7.19}$$

Integration of u over the cross-section gives the flow rate

$$Q = \frac{\pi R^2 A}{\rho c}(1 + \chi F) e^{i\omega t} = -\frac{\pi R^2}{i\omega\rho}(1 + \chi F)\frac{\partial p}{\partial z} \tag{7.20}$$

For the special case where the constraints are very strong, i.e. $K = -\infty$, it can be shown that

$$\frac{c}{c_0} = \frac{1 - F}{1 - \sigma^2} \tag{7.21}$$

Hence, for $\sigma = 0.5$, it follows from Eqs. (7.19) and (7.21)

$$\chi = -1 \tag{7.22}$$

or we have from Eq. (7.20)

$$-\frac{\partial p}{\partial z} = \frac{i\omega\rho}{\pi R^2}\frac{1}{1-F}Q \tag{7.23}$$

If we write

$$\frac{i\omega\rho}{\pi R^2}\frac{1}{1-F} = R_1 + i\omega L_1 \tag{7.24}$$

where R_1 and ωL_1 are the real and imaginary parts, Eq. (7.23) can be written as

$$-\frac{\partial p}{\partial z} = R_1 Q + L_1 \frac{\partial Q}{\partial t} \tag{7.25}$$

because Q varies with time as $\exp(i\omega t)$. Note that Eq. (7.25) is of the same form as the relationship between the electric current and time in an electric circuit with the resistance R_1, self-inductance L_1, and electromotive force $-\partial p/\partial z$.

An equation similar to Eq. (7.25) has also been derived:

$$-\frac{\partial Q}{\partial z} = Gp + C\frac{\partial p}{\partial t} \tag{7.26}$$

Here C is the compliance, analogous to electrical capacitance; the term Gp represents a seepage through the vessel walls proportional to the pressure; and G is the analogue of electrical shunt conductance.

Thurston (1973) showed that normal blood possesses viscoelastic properties. Since that time, attempts have been made to compare the observed pressure–flow relations for blood with the theory for oscillatory flow of a viscoelastic fluid. This has been done over a range of tube radii 0.0215–0.35 cm, and frequencies of oscillation 0.2–200 Hz. This fully covers the frequency range of physiological interest. The radii are comparable with those ranging from small arteries and veins up to the largest vessels. Thurston developed the theory of oscillatory flow of a linearly viscoelastic fluid in rigid circular tubes. His formula differs from that for a viscous fluid in that the Newtonian viscosity is replaced by the complex coefficient of viscosity $\eta^* = \eta' - i\eta''$. Thurston's study was limited to rigid

7.6 Pulsatile flow in microvessels

tubes; it would be better to extend the study to include the rheological properties of the vessel walls.

7.6 Pulsatile flow in microvessels

Until 1960, it was generally believed that pulsatile flow was unlikely, and that it did not occur in the microcirculation. However, Rappaport, Bloch & Irwin (1959) were able to measure fluctuating pressures in pulmonary arterioles; Gaehtgens (1970) observed significant pulsatile flow in the arterioles and venules of cat mesentery. Intaglietta, Richardson & Tompkins (1971) simultaneously measured pulsatile flow and pressure in the arterioles, capillaries and venules of cat omentum. As the pulse wave propagates through small vessels, the amplitude decreases, showing attenuation of the wave. Both pressure and velocity in microvessels show phase lag with respect to the arterial pressure.

The novel aspect of pulsatile flow in microvessels is that the non-Newtonian features of blood are most pronounced. Another pronounced feature is inhomogeneity, i.e. the existence of plasma layer near the vessel wall. The plasma layer can act as a 'lubricant' between the viscous core and the vessel's interior surface.

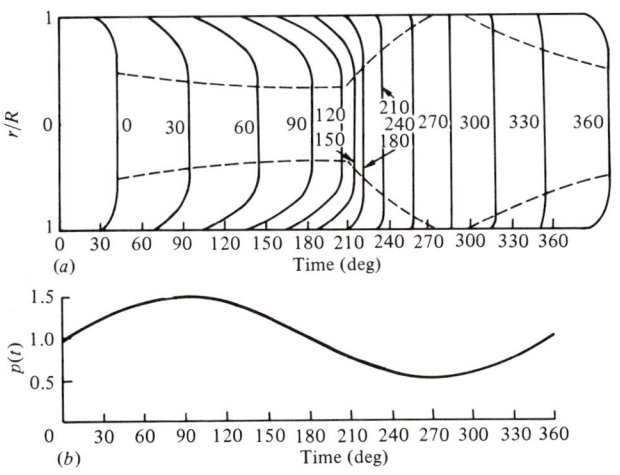

Fig. 70. (a) Velocity profiles of Casson fluid with plasma layer in a microvessel. (b) Pressure change during a cycle. (From Aroesty & Gross, 1972.)

Aroesty & Gross (1972) considered the experimental results on pulsatile flow in microvessels. They took into account the Casson fluid core with plasma layer in their theoretical study. Velocity profiles, at intervals of 30° in ωt, are shown in Fig. 70 for the indicated pressure gradient. The dashed lines indicate the yield surface, which separates plug and viscous flow. The location of a point where the yield stress is equal to the actual stress is called a yield point, and its locus is a yield surface.

Note that the pulsatile flow is assumed to be primarily a quasi-steady one. The yield stress of blood is probably related to rouleaux formation in the pressure of fibrinogen, and the time scale for the formation of rouleaux is assumed to be less than any flow time. Thus, the constitutive equation in unsteady flow is assumed to be identical with that in steady flow.

Horimoto, Koyama, Mishina & Asakura (1979) studied the velocity profiles in the arteriole (diameter 80 to 90 μm) of anaesthetized frog web by means of a laser Doppler microscope. Since the laser Doppler microscope yields a particle-biased mean of flow velocity, a method was postulated to estimate approximately the virtual velocity. The flow velocity at the central, median, and marginal portions as well as the pressure gradient along the stream axis varied in response to the cardiac cycle and with a certain time lag. The virtual velocity profile differed from the one predicted by the formula for a Newtonian fluid.

8

Hemorheological aspects of cardiovascular diseases

This chapter discusses the hemorheological aspects of cardiovascular diseases and their background – areas of rapid development in recent years.

8.1 Flow in a locally constricted tube

(a) *Steady flow*

Before we deal with the flow of a viscous fluid in a locally constricted tube, it is helpful to consider the steady laminar flow of an incompressible inviscid fluid. Such a flow is governed by Bernoulli's equation, which gives the relationship between velocity, pressure and elevation. Since there is assumed to be no viscous force, mechanical energy is conserved, and at any point on a streamline the following relationship holds:

$$p + \rho g h + \tfrac{1}{2}\rho v^2 = \text{const} \tag{8.1}$$

where p is the pressure, ρ is the density, g is the gravitational acceleration, h is the height, and v is the velocity. This is called *Bernoulli's equation*. Strictly speaking, it is not valid for blood flow, since blood is a viscous fluid.

Flow in a locally constricted vessel can be analysed theoretically using fluid mechanics. When streamlines are converging in the direction of flow, the fluid particles are accelerated, and the pressure drop becomes greater than that in a uniform tube. When the streamlines are diverging, the fluid particles are decelerated, and the pressure becomes smaller than that in a uniform tube, i.e. an adverse pressure gradient is expected. If the adverse pressure gradient becomes sufficiently large, it will cause the slowly moving fluid particles near the wall to reverse their directions of flow and a flow separation will occur (Fig. 71). The region which is surrounded by the dotted lines (surface) is called the *separation region*, where the fluid circulates and does not move downstream with the main stream; the dotted lines represent a streamline, and the upstream and downstream ends are called the *separation point* and the *reattachment point*, respectively. These points correspond to flow stagnation. These phenomena are known as *streamline separation*, or simply *separation*.

In the neighborhood of the separation point or the reattachment point, the fluid is almost in stasis and consequently the shear rate becomes very small. In blood flow, its viscosity will increase near these points due to the non-Newtonian shear-thinning behavior.

Forrester & Young (1970a, b) studied the steady laminar flow of a Newtonian fluid through an axisymmetric constricted tube. Since blood viscosity becomes independent of shear rate at shear rates above about 100 s^{-1} (see Sect. 3.4), blood can be considered as a Newtonian fluid, except possibly in particular regions where very low shear rates may occur. The axisymmetry is an assumption for mathematical simplicity. When the Reynolds number is not so large, the flow is laminar. Although arterial flow is pulsatile, the flow in small blood vessels may be regarded as quasi-steady at frequencies similar to those found in physiology, because the Womersley parameter α becomes very small.

In order to treat the problem, they limited themselves to a '*mild stenosis*'; the shape of the stenosis was sinusoidal, and the amplitude: wavelength ratio, δ/Z_0, was very small (Fig. 71). They took into account the nonlinear terms in the Navier–Stokes equation and obtained the approximate pressure gradient as follows:

$$-\frac{dp}{dz} = -\frac{5432}{1575\pi^2}\frac{\rho Q^2}{R^5}\frac{dR}{dz} + \frac{8\eta Q}{\pi R^4} \qquad (8.2)$$

Fig. 71. Velocity profiles and separation in a constricted tube. (From Forrester & Young, 1970a.)

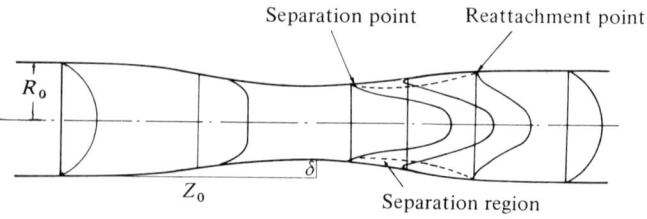

8.1 Flow in a locally constricted tube

where p is the pressure, Q is the flow rate, ρ is the density, and η is the viscosity of the fluid. In the above, z represents the distance along the axis in the direction of flow, the origin being the center of the stenosis; R is the radius of the tube at a point z. Note that Eq. (8.2) is reduced to Poiseuille's law in the particular case of a uniform tube. In a constricted tube, the pressure gradient consists of two terms. The first term represents the contribution due to the inertia of the fluid, and the second term the contribution due to the viscosity of the fluid. In the converging portion of the tube ($z < 0$), dR/dz is negative, so that the inertia term increases the pressure drop. But in the diverging portion ($z > 0$), dR/dz is positive, so that an adverse pressure gradient ($dp/dz > 0$) develops. This contributes to the presence of the backward in the separation region.

A dimensionless form of the pressure drop from the upstream end of the stenosis ($z = -Z_0$), where $p = p_0$, to any position along the stenosis can be obtained by integrating Eq. (8.2). The result is shown in Fig. 72. The dashed curves represent the dimensionless pressure drops for Poiseuille flow.

Forrester & Young (1970a) further found that the wall shear stress τ_w was approximated by

$$\frac{\tau_w}{\rho U_0^2} = -\frac{616}{1575}\frac{R_0^4}{R^4}\frac{dR}{dz} + \frac{8}{Re_0}\frac{R_0^3}{R^3} \qquad (8.3)$$

where R_0 is the radius of the tube far away from the constriction,

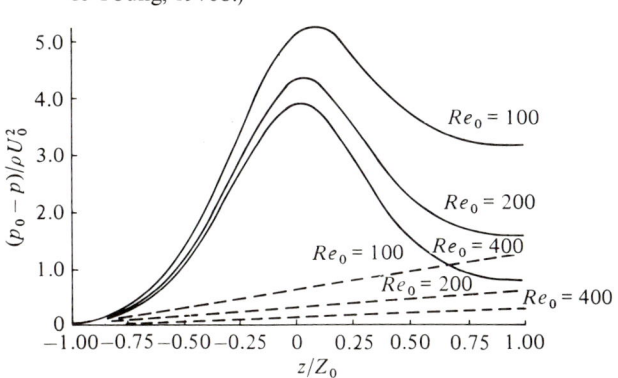

Fig. 72. Pressure drop along the constriction. (From Forrester & Young, 1970b.)

U_0 and Re_0 are, respectively, the average velocity and the Reynolds number far away from the constriction.

Lee & Fung (1971) specified the geometry of the constriction as a bell-shaped curve given by the equation:

$$\frac{r}{R_0} = 1 - b \exp\left(-\frac{cz^2}{R_0^2}\right) \tag{8.4}$$

where R_0 is the radius of the tube far away from the origin, b is the amplitude of the local constriction ($b > 0$), and c is the sharpness factor. A larger value of c means a sharper profile, whereas a smaller value means a flatter profile. Thus, they dealt with a mild and a *sharp stenosis*. A detailed picture is presented of the distributions of velocity, pressure, and shear stress on the wall. The flow pattern calculated for the Reynolds number $Re_0 = 25$ is shown in Fig. 73.

If we write the wall shear stress τ_w in the form

$$\tau_w = -\eta \frac{2U_0}{R_0} \Omega_w \tag{8.5}$$

then Ω_w means a dimensionless wall shear stress. Figure 74 shows the distribution of Ω_w for three Reynolds numbers, $Re_0 = 1, 10$, and 25. At a large distance from the constriction, the dimensionless wall shear stress Ω_w tends to 2, which is the value for a Poiseuille flow. Note that the distribution of wall shear stress is asymmetric, and that the site of the maximum wall shear stress shifts a little upstream with respect to the line $z = 0$, as is expected.

The profile of a tube with a local dilation can be specified by taking negative values of b. Contrary to the flow in a constricted

Fig. 73. Streamlines in a constricted tube. (From Lee & Fung, 1971.)

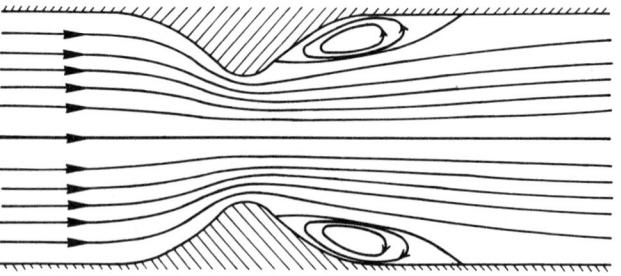

8.1 Flow in a locally constricted tube

tube, no eddy appears in the dilated region in the case of $b = -0.4$, $c = 4$, and $Re_0 = 25$. The maximum wall shear stress is only slightly larger than that of a Poiseuille flow.

(b) Pulsatile flow

Pulsatile flow through a tube with a constriction is very complex; experiments using models are helpful. Young & Tsai (1973) used hot-film measurements to investigate the development of turbulence, and they found that in a mildly constricted model the critical Reynolds number was considerably larger than the corresponding value for steady flow. In more severely constricted models the critical Reynolds number for oscillatory flow was a little lower than that for steady flow.

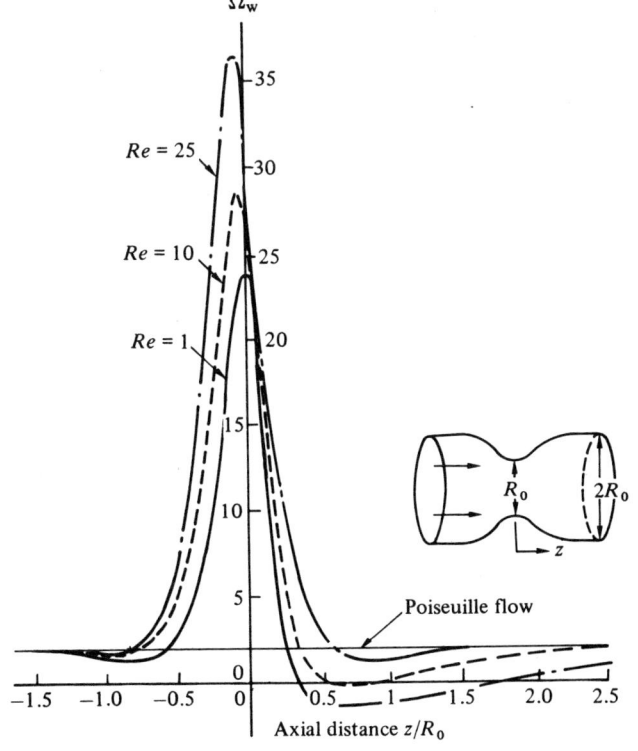

Fig. 74. Distribution of wall shear stress in a constricted tube. (From Lee & Fung, 1971.)

Hemorheological aspects of cardiovascular diseases 156

Fig. 75. Steady and pulsatile flow in a constricted tube. (From Azuma & Fukushima, 1976.)

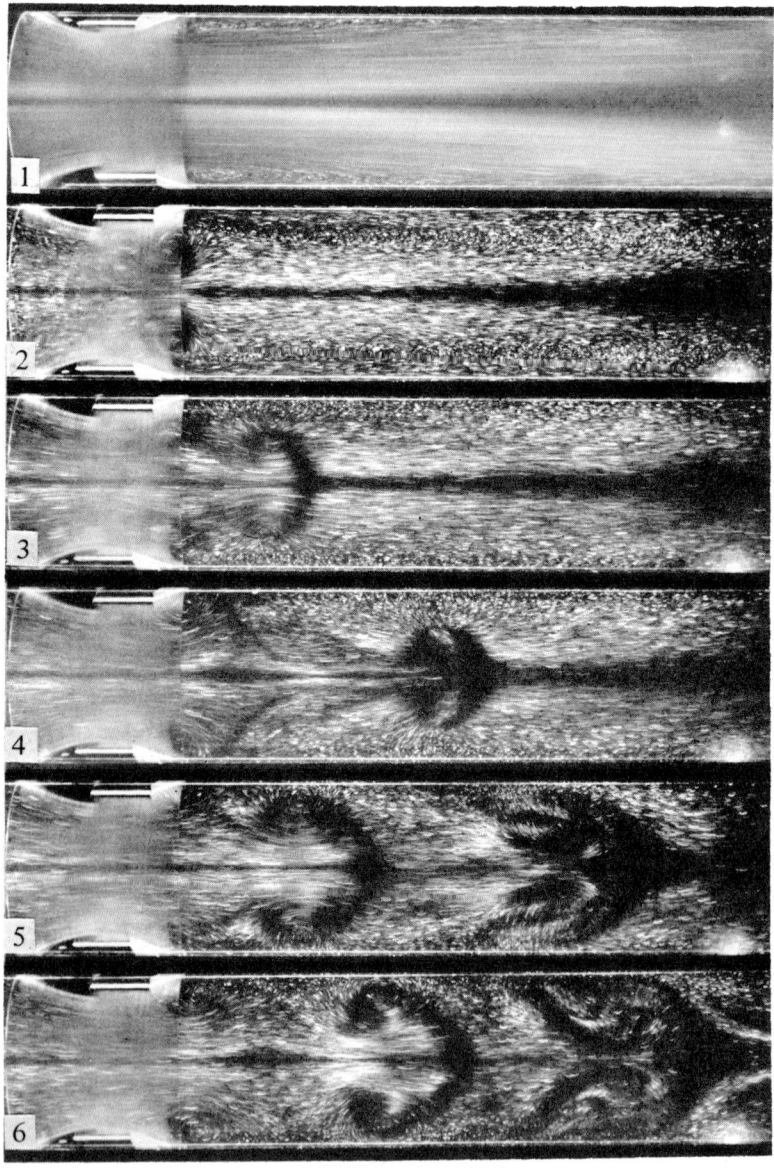

Azuma & Fukushima (1976) studied the steady and pulsatile flows in stenotic blood vessel models. Both axisymmetric and non-axisymmetric models, having different diameter ratios of constriction, were used in the experiments. The flow patterns, visualized by the aluminium dust method, are shown in Fig. 75. The presence of an axisymmetric constriction caused pulsatile disturbances. Azuma & Fukushima (1976) found that, as the acceleration increased, large vortices were formed near the constriction, shed downstream and broken down into turbulence. The turbulent flow thus formed did not diminish during the decelerating phase, but spread upstream against the flow direction until the start of the next accelerating phase. Pulsation seems to facilitate not only the production of vortices, but also the backward spread of turbulence formed downstream.

8.2 Post-stenotic dilatation

Dilatation of the arterial wall distal to a constriction is a common clinical finding. This frequently occurs in the ascending aorta above a stenotic aortic valve, and also distal to atherosclerotic lesions; it is called *post-stenotic dilatation*.

There are several theories about what causes post-stenotic dilatation. They may be classified as follows:

(a) *Turbulence theory*

If the constriction is so severe that turbulence is generated, it is quite likely that fluctuating pressures and tangential stresses on the endothelial lining may cause a deterioration of the endothelial cells. This could lead to subsequent degeneration and weakening of the arterial wall, which in turn causes post-stenotic dilatation.

(b) *Separation theory*

In the separation region downstream from a stenosis, deterioration and weakening of the arterial wall may occur due to an insufficient supply of nutrients and oxygen. This theory is based on the assumption that the exchange of substances between the separation region and the main stream of flow is relatively small. It should be noted that a practically stagnant region never exists in pulsatile flow.

(c) **Pressure theory**

This theory assumes that the pressure in the diverging portion of a stenosis is the cause of post-stenotic dilatation. As is seen in Fig. 72, the pressure in the diverging portion is at a lower level than that upstream. Thus, the post-stenotic dilatation cannot be explained by this theory.

(d) **Shear stress theory**

This theory assumes that the wall shear stress in the diverging portion is the cause of post-stenotic dilatation. Since in steady flow the wall shear stress in the diverging portion is generally smaller than that in the converging portion of the stenosis, shear stress is unlikely to cause post-stenotic dilatation.

Matunobu & Arakawa (1974) studied the effect of the wall shear stress in pulsatile flow using a simple model of a blood vessel with a stenosis, i.e. a transparent conduit with rectangular cross-section and a plane barrier fitted perpendicularly to the bottom. They performed experiments with the degrees of stenosis (the ratio of effective height of the stenosis to that of the conduit) 0.30, 0.55 and 0.74, the pulse frequencies 0.5, 1.0 and 2.0 Hz, and the flow rate 0.33 ℓ min^{-1}. They allowed starch to settle evenly on the bottom of the conduit before water was pumped through it. They found that the starch layer was eroded near the mean position of the stagnation, and further that its rate increased with the frequency of pulsation and the degree of stenosis. The wall shear stress may have played an important role in the post-stenotic phenomena for the starch layer. But no quantitative conclusion was reached.

8.3 Flow at branching sites

Flow structure at branching sites is of particular interest with respect to the hemodynamic mechanism of atherogenesis, discussed in later sections. Kandarpa & Davids (1976) analysed the steady laminar flow of an incompressible Newtonian fluid in a symmetrically bifurcated channel using the finite element method. They assumed that the cross-section of the channel was rectangular, and the wall was rigid and impermeable. They also assumed laminar flow, since it is doubtful whether turbulence occurs in smaller mammals (for example dogs). The calculated velocity profiles are

8.3 Flow at branching sites

shown in Fig. 76. It can be seen that the input profile develops normally in the straight segment, but that at a short distance into the tapered segment, along the outer wall, boundary layer separation and backflow appear. The backflow region extends into a portion of the branch. As the flow proceeds down the branch, a parabolic profile is re-established.

Niimi *et al.* (1976) observed steady and pulsatile flow patterns in bifurcations, using the flow-visualization method in the model experiments. Figure 77 shows the steady flow pattern for a Reynolds number of about 1 300 with respect to the main tube. Similar to the flow in the bifurcated channel, flow separation occurs. Moreover, a

Fig. 76. Velocity profile in a symmetrically bifurcated channel. (From Kandarpa & Davids, 1976.)

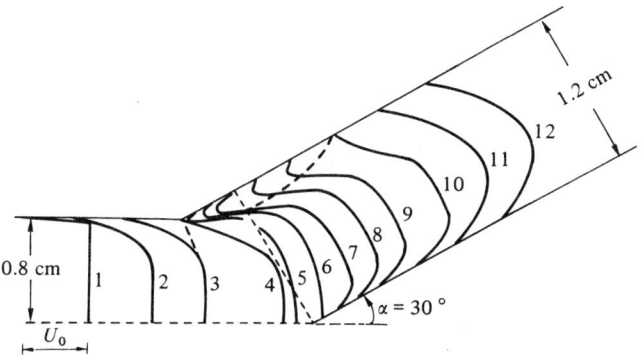

Fig. 77. Steady flow pattern in a bifurcated tube. (From Niimi et al., 1976.)

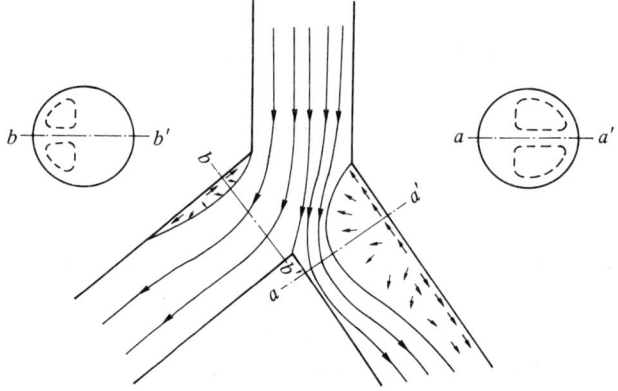

pair of vortices are induced in the cross-sections $a-a'$ and $b-b'$; these are the so-called secondary flows due to the curvature of the main stream; the fluid flows helically through the distal branches. They found that as the Reynolds number increases, the vortices are distorted and shed downstream. They further found that in pulsatile flow the flow separation and the vortices are generated and shed downstream periodically. It should be noted that a practically stagnant region does not exist in pulsatile flow.

Karino, Kwong & Goldsmith (1979) studied the flow patterns in glass models of 3 mm diameter, which had right-angled T-junctions with square or rounded corners. They took cine films of the paths of micro-spheres in dilute suspensions at inflow Reynolds numbers, Re_0, from 15 to 420, and flow ratios Q_1/Q_2 for the main: side tubes from 0.05 to 4.0. In the square T-junction, paired vortices symmetrical about the common median plane formed at the entrances of the main and side daughter tubes over a wide range of Re_0 and Q_1/Q_2; in the rounded T-junction, the main vortex was formed at a lower, and the side vortex at a higher Re_0 than in the square T-junction. When flow entered the side tube, paired connected vortices were also formed, but only when one daughter tube was severely occluded.

8.4 Thrombosis

When blood coagulates in a blood vessel *in vivo*, the process is generally called '*thrombosis*'. Since the terms 'thrombosis' and '*thrombus*' are often used interchangeably, it must be emphasized that these terms are not synonyms (Copley, 1979).

The occurrence of a thrombus or numerous thrombi can be entirely physiological. It does not necessarily progress and become a pathological condition with or without clinical manifestations. However, 'thrombus' usually means a pathological condition which may have clinical manifestations.

Sometimes the stresses exerted by blood flowing past a thrombus may cause the thrombus to break away. This is then carried through the vascular system until it plugs a smaller blood vessel. Such a thrombus is called '*embolus*'. The condition in which a vessel is occluded by an embolus is called '*embolism*'.

The process of thrombosis differs in fact at different sites in the

8.4 Thrombosis

circulation. This is probably due to the strong influence of the local flow condition. Furthermore, the structure of thrombi not only differs from that of clots, but it may also be different in different parts in the blood circulation. This may be due to the fact that the initiating mechanism of thrombosis is usually somewhat different from that of clotting, and that thrombus formation is always subjected to fluid-mechanical influences. Thus hemorheology is very important in the study of thrombosis.

The detailed mechanism of thrombus formation is not yet clear. There are multiple causes of thrombosis, and the process can occur anywhere in the blood circulation in different ways.

Thrombi, like clots, consist of various elements of blood trapped in a fibrin mesh-work. But the initiating mechanism of thrombosis is usually somewhat different. In arteries, at least, the crucial initial event is the formation of an aggregate of platelets, on which layers of fibrin and blood cells are subsequently deposited.

Under normal conditions platelets do not adhere to one another or to vessel walls, due to the repulsion of their like charges. A major role is ascribed to ADP (adenosine diphosphate) as an initiator of platelet aggregation and adhesion to the endothelium, in the presence of a hydrodynamic collision mechanism. ADP is released from platelets as well as damaged red cells and connective tissue (collagen) at sites of injury.

Let us take a brief look at blood clotting. A blood clot consists of a mesh of fibrin, and red and white cells and platelets entangled in this mesh. Fibrin formation involves a complicated series of enzymatic reactions. The basic clotting process may be described as follows: release of thromboplastin → prothrombin to thrombin → fibrinogen to fibrin → polymerization of fibrin fibers → formation of clot.

Copley (1974) distinguished three major processes of blood clotting and thrombus formation: (i) non-enzymatic fibrinogen aggregation; (ii) blood cellular clumping; (iii) thrombin-induced fibrin coagulation (Fig. 78). He emphasized that thrombus formation can only begin after the aggregation of fibrinogen molecules. The inner surface of blood vessels is lined with endothelial fibrin, to which fibrinogen molecules attach.

Let us now discuss hemorheological aspects of thrombosis.

(a) *Turbulence and thrombosis*

Mitchell and Schwartz (1965) suggested that turbulence causes thrombosis by damaging both the blood and the arterial wall.

According to Smith, Blick, Coalson & Stein (1972) and Stein & Sabbah (1974), not only does turbulence contribute to thrombus formation, but the size of clot formed also seems to be directly proportional to the intensity of the turbulence, which, in turn, is directly proportional to the Reynolds number. Consequently, for a given flow rate, vessels with smaller radii may have an increased propensity to form thromboses.

(b) *Stasis and thrombosis*

Theories that stasis favors thrombosis have been put forward by several investigators. Fox & Hugh (1966) suggested that thrombosis is more often associated with areas of stasis. Blood vessel walls adjacent to areas of stasis may have lesions due to some metabolic disorder.

Merrill *et al.* (Merrill, Cokelet, Britten & Wells, 1963; Merrill, Gilliland, Lee & Salzman, 1966) suggested that structures might develop between red blood cells and fibrinogen molecules in regions of stagnant or nearly stagnant flow near the vessel wall. Thrombus formation could develop if fibrinogen is converted to fibrin.

The above view was supported by Fry (1973). He suggested that the concentration of fibrinogen might increase between the blood and the blood vessel wall, since fibrinogen is not so hydrophilic.

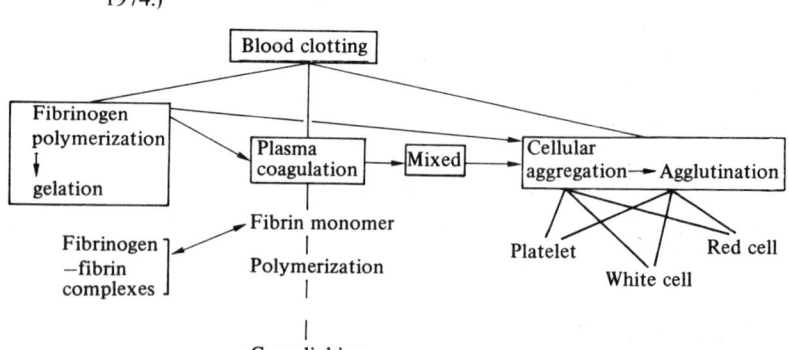

Fig. 78. Three major processes of blood clotting. (From Copley, 1974.)

Thus a fibrin network might develop in the stagnant blood near the separation and reattachment points.

Dintenfass (1964) stated that aggregation of red cells increased at low shear rates. This may also happen with thrombus formation in or near separation regions.

8.5 Atherosclerosis

(a) *A general description*

Atherosclerosis is a disease mainly of the inner layers of the arteries. Its importance as a major cause of myocardial and cerebral infarction and thrombosis has been appreciated for many years. This disease develops over a long period before symptoms appear, and consists mainly of three stages, i.e. an initial or early stage, a mid-stage, and a late stage. It is difficult to follow the early development of the disease in individual patients. In addition, atherosclerosis is a multifactor disease. Much clinical research has involved risk factors, especially hyperlipidemia and hypertension. Nevertheless, its pathogenesis is not well understood.

In its early stages, atherosclerosis is manifested by local deposition of lipid on the interface between blood and the arterial wall (endothelial surface), or just within the intima. The major role of lipid metabolism in *atherogenesis* has been pointed out by many investigators. The metabolic theory of atherogenesis focuses on reduced enzyme activity as its key feature. For instance, Adams & Bayliss (1969) suggested that intimal thickening reduces oxygen flow to medial enzyme sites, thereby reducing enzyme activity.

Ross & Glomset (1976), and others studied the role of smooth-muscle cell proliferation in lesion formation. Fundamental research into factors that control cell proliferation will be essential for understanding atherogenesis. Atherosclerosis may result from an endothelial injury, which may have different manifestations in different sites in different arteries. The injury may produce, through metabolic processes, similar alterations in endothelium and smooth muscle which in turn cause the smooth-muscle proliferation, excessive connective-tissue formation and lipid deposition that we call atherosclerosis.

Although endothelial injury is an important aspect of atherogenesis, so are hemodynamic factors.

(b) *Hemodynamic theories*

The question of why atherosclerotic lesions tend to occur in particular places has long been discussed by many investigators. Usually, atherosclerotic plaques occur at particular sites in arteries where abrupt changes in the vessel geometry occur, for example at curvatures or at entrances of branching vessels. Various hemodynamic or hemorheological theories have been proposed to correlate the favored sites with local flow conditions in the arterial system.

Let us summarize briefly the hemodynamic theories discussed by Gessner (1973). Common areas in the major central arteries include the inner wall of a curved segment, the proximal lip of a branch, and the lateral walls of the aortic–iliac bifurcation. The flow region adjacent to these sites is generally a separation region of low shear rate, or a turbulent region. Also, lesions can develop in regions of relatively high wall shear stress, such as those near the distal lip of a branch, and along the medial walls of the aortic–iliac bifurcation. The hemodynamic theories may be classified into the following broad categories:

(i) Pressure theory

Texon, Imparato & Helpern (1965) proposed that suction on the endothelium surface causes damage to the endothelium and the adjacent wall layers, with subsequent thickening of the intima and eventual plaque development. Since it is unlikely that negative transmural pressure is ever generated across the walls of an artery for any significant period of time, this theory is untenable.

Hypertension is a cause of atherosclerosis. The effect of high blood pressure on vascular permeability will be referred to later.

(ii) Turbulence theory

Some atherosclerotic sites correspond to anticipated regions of local turbulence. Mitchell & Schwartz (1965) suggest that turbulent velocity and pressure fluctuations at branching sites cause platelets to be damaged and eventually form mural thrombi or elevated plaques on the intima. Wesolowski, Fries, Sabin & Sawyer (1965) suggest that atherosclerotic lesions can develop in regions of turbulence as a result of induced vibration in the arterial wall or local increases in lateral wall pressure.

The validity of these theories depends on whether turbulent

wall pressure fluctuations are of sufficient magnitude to cause any injury to the arterial wall; Fry showed experimentally that a high intensity of turbulent fluctuations enhances vascular permeability to serum albumin.

In view of the possible contribution of turbulent flow to atherogenesis, particularly at bifurcations of vessels, Stein, Sabbah, Anbe & Walburn (1979) measured the flow velocity in the abdominal aorta and common iliac artery in eight resting patients, using a hot-film velocimeter. The peak Reynolds number, measured at the aortic bifurcation (in four patients), ranged from 400 to 1100, and in the common iliac artery it ranged from 390 to 620. Absence of turbulent flow in the abdominal aorta and common iliac arteries in resting patients suggests that turbulence does not initiate atherosclerosis in these areas. However, it is possible that turbulence contributes to atherosclerosis, once plaque formation has caused an irregularity in the arterial walls.

(iii) Flow separation theory

Fox & Hugh (1966) suggested that blood stream stagnates locally in the separation region, and that this allows platelets and fibrin to form a mesh at the wall in which lipid particles become trapped and eventually coalesce to form atheromatous plaques. It should be noted that in pulsatile flow no such quiescent region can exist. According to Chien, (1976) the 'dwell-time' of a platelet in the vicinity of an endothelial surface is a function of the local velocity gradient. Areas of low shear and areas of flow separation have particularly long 'dwell-time' as compared to regions of high shear, suggesting that if platelet–endothelial interaction occurs, it is more likely in low shear areas.

(iv) Shear stress theory

Fry suggested the deformation, swelling, and eventual erosion of the endothelium may occur where the local wall shear stress is relatively high. He showed experimentally that the wall shear stress enhances vascular permeability to serum albumin, and that exposure of the endothelial surface to a time-averaged wall shear stress of approximately 380 dyn cm^{-2} resulted in marked deterioration of the endothelial surface. He also demonstrated that shear rates substantially below these critical values can nevertheless cause increased albumin transfer through the intima. Nakache &

Péronneau (1979) admit that, even at shear rates below those at which endothelial damage appears, an increased flow of lipoproteins to and from the wall exists.

In contrast, Caro, Pedley, Schroter & Seed (1978) indicated that early lesions tend to develop predominantly in regions of low wall shear stress, for example in the terminal abdominal aorta just proximal to the aortic–iliac bifurcation and near the proximal lip of a branch. Possible reasons for the differing results were discussed by Caro *et al.* based on a *mass transfer boundary layer*, across which the concentration of solute varies from its value in the core of the artery to its value at the wall. It was hypothesized that the development of early lesions is related to locally reduced efflux of accumulating material, from wall to blood, due to locally reduced wall shear rate. The presence of the thin boundary layer of high concentration of solute is considered to be responsible for the locally reduced efflux. However, the theory proposed by Caro admits the possibility of rapid development of lesions in the areas with a high shear rate, when there is high concentration of blood cholesterol. Thus, Fry's hypothesis is also admitted by Caro under certain circumstances.

Fig. 79. Processes in early development of atheroma. (From Copley, 1979.)

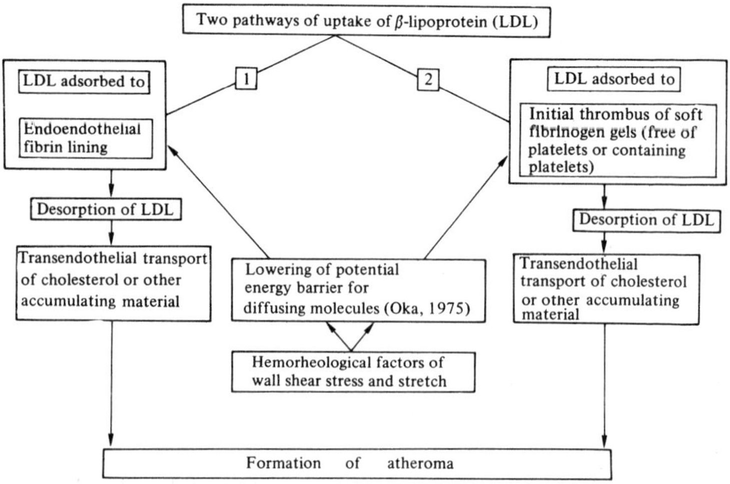

(c) Surface chemical theory

Copley (1979) drew attention to the role of the interface between the wall and blood in atherogenesis. His theory is concerned with the early development of atheroma, and proposes two ways of uptake of low density lipoprotein (LDL). They are: on the endothelial fibrin lining; and on fibrinogen gels, loosely structured due to an action of LDL which he discovered. His theory also incorporates the present writer's theory concerning hemorheology and other physical factors. The theory is furthermore based on surface chemical findings by Miller, Graet & Frei (1973), who studied cholesterol exchange between surface layers and plasma proteins in bulk. Their findings suggest that lipoproteins, which transport cholesterol, can adsorb reversibly on a proteinous surface. Copley's theory is shown diagrammatically in Fig. 79.

8.6 Protein uptake by arterial wall

Experimental studies on protein uptake by the arterial wall have been put forward by many investigators, including Fry

Fig. 80. Effect of shear stress and turbulence on albumin uptake by aortic wall. τ: Shear stress, p: pressure, I: intensity of transmitted light, i: turbulence intensity, A: plug entrance, B: plug exit. (From Fry, 1969.)

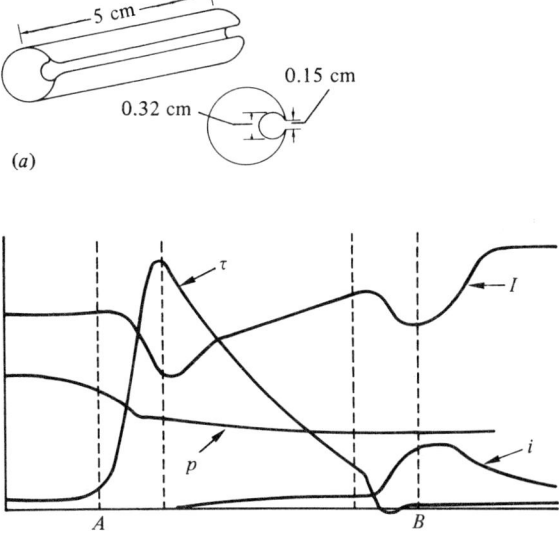

(1973) and Nerem, Mosberg & Schwerin (1976). In order to examine the relationship of the flow field to the protein uptake by the arterial wall, Fry inserted a plug with a narrow longitudinal channel along its surface into the descending thoracic aorta of dogs (Fig. 80(a)). Blood in the region upstream of the plug would accelerate into the small channel and decelerate just downstream of the end of the plug. The rapid flow within the channel would exert high shear stresses on the endothelial surface. The exit region would show low shear stress, but turbulent eddies would set up there.

Fry intravenously injected Evans blue dye, which formed a stable chemical complex with serum albumin; any increase in endothelial stain indicated increased transport of serum albumin to the endothelial surface. He measured the deposition of serum albumin by

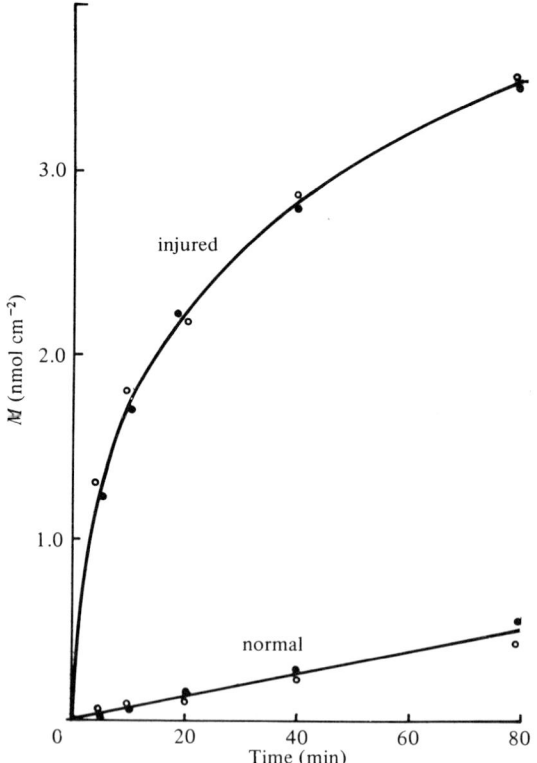

Fig. 81. Surface concentration of albumin in arterial wall as a function of time. (From Fry, 1973.)

8.6 Protein uptake by arterial wall

photometric means. Fig. 80(b) shows a typical set of experimental results. It can be seen that the flux of serum albumin to the endothelial surface is enhanced by large shear stress as well as by a high intensity of turbulence.

Fry also measured the surface concentration M of dye, i.e. serum albumin uptake by arterial wall, as a function of time (Fig. 81). In the figure, M increases in proportion to time on a normal surface; the upper curve is for an injured surface, the endothelial cells having been gently damaged with a wet brush of camel's hair. Thus, even a normal endothelial surface provides a significant energy barrier to the transport of albumin. The amount of albumin transported is not appreciably affected by the transmural pressure on either a normal or an injured surface. This suggests that, for albumin transport, pressure is ineffective and that diffusive forces predominate.

Carew (1973) studied the effect of the shear stress due to the adjacent flow on the transport of albumin across the endothelial surface *in vitro*. Figure 82 shows that the excess surface concentration is proportional to the wall shear stress squared. The elastic energy stored in an elastic surface deformed in shear varies with τ^2. This is consistent with Fry's suggestion that if energy is supplied to the vascular surface, its permeability to protein appears to increase.

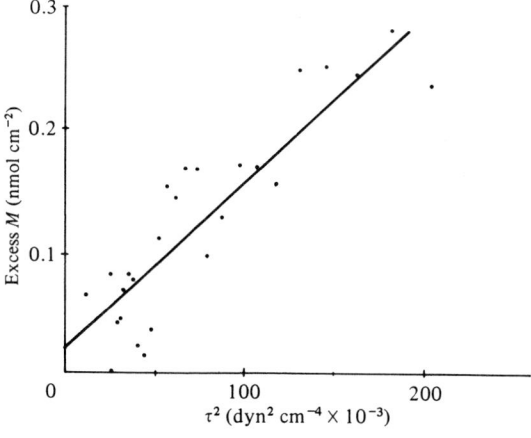

Fig. 82. Surface concentration of albumin vs. wall shear stress squared. (From Carew, 1971.)

Fry studied the effect of increased wall stretch on the excess surface concentration of albumin (Fig. 83). If stretch λ is defined as the stretched dimension of the surface divided by its unstretched dimension, a normal physiological stretch is about 1.4.

Nerem *et al.* measured *in vitro* the uptake of ^{131}I-albumin by the

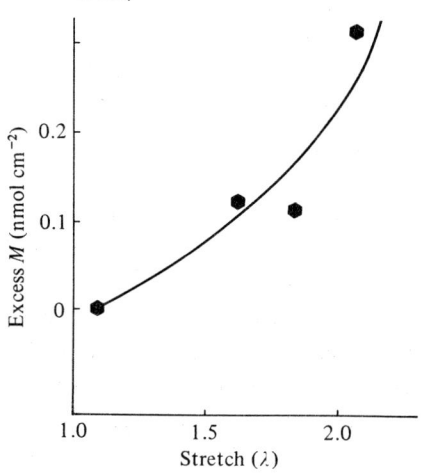

Fig. 83. Excess uptake of albumin vs. stretch ratio λ. (From Fry, 1973.)

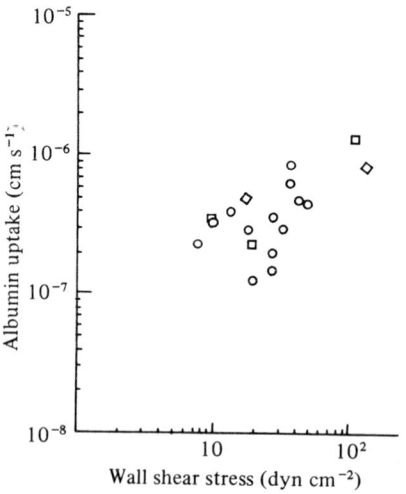

Fig. 84. Albumin uptake vs. wall shear stress. ○ Serum, 100mm Hg; □ Serum, 10mm Hg; ◊ blood, 10mm Hg. (From Nerem *et al.*, 1976.)

arterial wall in a dog's serum-perfused common carotid artery and aorta. The results of the steady-state in-vitro perfusion experiments demonstrate a slight shear dependence of $\tau_w^{0.38}$ (Fig. 84).

They also performed *in vitro* sinusoidally oscillating flow perfusion experiments on excised dog common carotid arteries. For data obtained at a peak wall shear stress of less than approximately 50 dyn cm^{-2}, the uptake shows the shear dependence on $\tau_w^{0.5}$. This weak dependence is consistent with the steady-state in-vitro perfusion results mentioned above.

Furthermore, they performed *wholebody vibration* experiments at 10 Hz and a peak-to-peak amplitude of 1.27 cm. ^{131}I-albumin uptake by the arterial wall at the posterior ascending aorta site is on average double that of the non-vibration data.

8.7 Permeability and pathways of macromolecules

(a) Permeability

Let us consider mass transport across a membrane. Its fundamental mechanisms are diffusion and convection. When a substance is transported in a direction x, the number of moles per unit time passing through a plane perpendicular to the direction x is usually called the *molar flux*. In the mass transport across artery walls, diffusion is much more important than convection. The molar flux is here considered on the basis of Fick's law:

$$J = -DA \, dc/dx \tag{8.6}$$

where dc/dx is the concentration gradient of the substance in the direction x, D is the diffusion coefficient, and A is the cross-sectional areas across which transport takes place. Note that c is measured in the units of mol cm^{-3}, D in the units cm^2 s^{-1}, and J in the units mol s^{-1}.

In the diffusion through a cell membrane, the permeability is conveniently defined by

$$P = D/\Delta x \tag{8.7}$$

where Δx is the thickness of the membrane. Then P is measured in the units cm s^{-1}. If we denote the difference between the concentrations on both sides of the membrane by Δc, and the effective area of the membrane available for transport by A, then we have from

Eq. (8.6):

$$J = PA \Delta c \tag{8.8}$$

The simplest model of a biological membrane can be regarded as porous, with the size and density of the pores governing the diffusion through the membrane. Although both the thickness and effective area of the membrane are usually unknown, the *permeability area product*, PA, can be obtained from the experimentally derivable quantities J and Δc.

Both the permeability, P, and the effective area, A, depend on the molecular weight, i.e. the molecular size of the substance. The capillary permeability area product for polyvinyl pyrrolidone is plotted against the molecular weight in Fig. 85, indicating that there are different transport mechanisms for small and large molecules across the capillary membrane.

If we take into account the effect of convection, Eq. (8.8) is replaced by

$$J = PA \Delta c + J_v(1 - \sigma)\bar{c} \tag{8.9}$$

where J_v is the convective flux, σ is the solute reflection coefficient, and $\bar{c}$ is the mean solute concentration in the convective channels. In the above, the second term stands for the convective term.

(b) *Diffusion coefficient*

Diffusion is caused by the random Brownian motion of

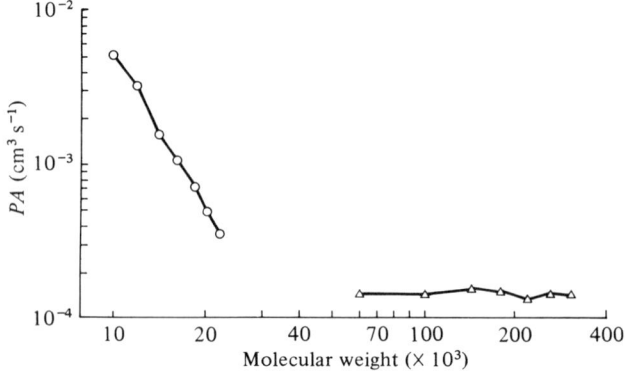

Fig. 85. Capillary permeability area product vs. molecular weight. (From Renkin, 1964.)

molecules; the diffusion coefficient D is temperature dependent and is given by

$$D = kT/f \tag{8.10}$$

where T is the absolute temperature, k is Boltzmann's constant, and f is the frictional constant of the molecule.

In the theory of rate processes, the elementary process of diffusion is understood to be the jump of a molecule from one equilibrium position to the next, over a potential barrier; the diffusion coefficient is usually expressed within a small range of temperatures:

$$D = A \exp(-E/RT) \tag{8.11}$$

where E is the *activation energy for diffusion*, R is the gas constant, and A is a constant.

(c) *Junctions*

The innermost surface of blood vessels is always lined with endothelium. Several pathways for endothelial transport of material have been proposed, and are classified into three categories: (i) direct pathway through the endothelial cells; (ii) passage along *junctions* between endothelial cells; (iii) active transport by *vesicles* through a process called *pinocytosis*. The pathways depend not only upon the nature of the material transported, but also upon the regions of arteries and capillaries, and upon whether they are in a normal or inflamed state. The electron microscope has made a great contribution to the study of the pathways.

The width of a junction is usually about 15–20 nm. But there is localized narrow site called the *junctional complex*, about 8 nm wide, approximately one third of the way along a junction from the luminal surface (Fig. 86). A so-called '*tight junction*' forms a continuous band around the side of the cells, and large molecules cannot pass through it. In a so-called '*spot welded junction*', large molecules may pass through it.

Karnowsky (1967) produced electron microscopic evidence that when peroxidase with a molecular weight of 40 000 is injected intravenously it can be found along the entire length of the junction in the mouse myocardium, diaphragm, and gastrocnemius.

In addition, electron microscopic studies have demonstrated very distinctive differences in the structure of capillaries in various specialized tissues of the body. Simionescu and his co-workers (1975) showed that the anatomically tight junctions in various tissues differ in permeability. This suggests that there are important distinctions in the microstructures of anatomically tight junctions.

Wissig (1979) showed that the structures of endothelial junctions of capillaries and post-capillary venules of muscle differ. The permeability of these vessels to protein is related to structural features in their endothelial junctions. Particularly with regard to venules, other factors in addition to the structure of their endothelial junctions may regulate the movement of protein across their endothelium.

(d) Vesicles

Palade & Bruns (1968) proposed vesicles as a transport system across the endothelium. There are about 500 vesicles per cell. Two types of vesicles can be distinguished; free vesicles, and attached vesicles. Free vesicles exist within the cytoplasm of the cells; they are nearly spherical, 60–80 nm in diameter. A vesicle

Fig. 86. Endothelial junctions. (From Caro *et al.*, 1978.)

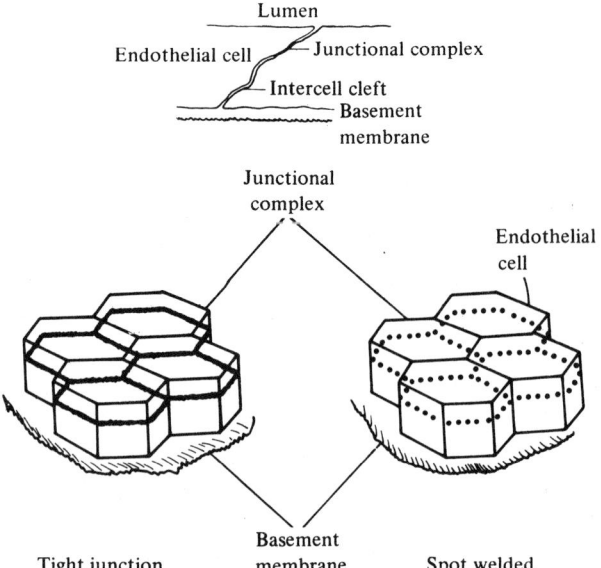

8.8 Vascular permeability to proteins

attached to cell membrane becomes open to the exterior of the cell and forms a neck, about 25 nm in length (Fig. 87).

The motion of free vesicles is thought to be due to the Brownian motion of the vesicles. The detailed mechanism of interaction between attached vesicles and cell membrane is not yet clear. Since the neck of the attached vesicles is rather narrow, large molecules with diameter greater than about 50 nm cannot be transported by vesicles.

Electron microscopic studies indicate that horseradish peroxidase enters the wall both via the intercellular junctions and the endothelial vesicles, whereas ferritin and lactoperoxidase enter only via the vesicles.

8.8 Physical theory of vascular permeability to proteins

Hemorheological studies of atherogenesis have produced physical theories to explain the uptake of serum albumin by arterial walls. No experiments have yet determined the pathways of serum albumin across the endothelial surface of arteries, but it is more likely that vesicular transport is involved rather than the intercellular junctions, because the diameter of the serum albumin molecule is 7 nm while the gap within the junctional complex, the narrowest site in the intercellular cleft, is thought to be approximately 8 nm wide.

(a) *A molecular picture of protoplasm*

Seifriz (1924) inserted a nickel particle into the interior of a

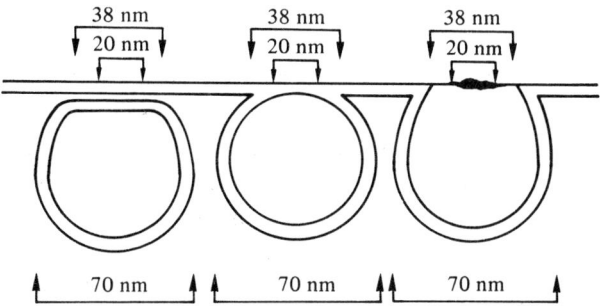

Fig. 87. Interaction between a vesicle and the cell membrane. (From Palade & Bruns, 1968.)

cell and caused it to move by applying a magnetic field with an electromagnet. When the nickel particle was in the *endoplasm* of the cell, it moved comparatively freely and did not return to its original position when the current was cut off from the magnet. Thus, the endoplasm was considered as having viscosity. But when the nickel particle was in the *cortex*, it returned to its original position when the current was shut off, indicating elasticity of the cortex.

Many investigators later showed that the viscosity of *protoplasm* is non-Newtonian. In fact, Kamiya & Kuroda (1958) showed it for the protoplasm of myxomycete plasmodium. Hiramoto (1969, 1970) also studied the rheological properties of the protoplasm of sea urchin eggs by the *magnetic particle method*, and determined the viscoelasticity of the protoplasm. Seifriz showed that the nickel particle in the cortex moved more freely when a magnetic field was applied intermittently and repeatedly. This indicates that protoplasm exhibits thixotropy, i.e. isothermal reversible change from gel to sol is produced by mechanical disturbance.

If we consider the peculiar rheological properties of protoplasm, such as non-Newtonian viscosity, viscoelasticity, and thixotropy, we can draw the following molecular picture of protoplasm in endothelial cells.

A number of bonds must exist between polar or ionized groups of protein molecules. In fact, 50% of the dry weight of living matter is protein. The bonds are thought to be van der Waals bonds, which are rather strong in general. However, they must be relatively weak in our case since protoplasm exhibits thixotropy. This conclusion also has theoretical support, if we remember that polar groups are hydrated and that ionized groups are electrically shielded by counter ions.

Since the van der Waals bonds with which we are here concerned are relatively weak, they may be broken down by external forces to some extent, depending upon their magnitude and duration. This molecular picture certainly corresponds to the thixotropic behavior of protoplasm. Consequently, it can be expected that any external disturbance causing breakdown of bonds will lower the viscosity and facilitate the vesicular transport through the protoplasm of endothelial cells. It has hitherto been thought that the passage of large molecules such as protein molecules required large pores, which would briefly open and close. In place of this is a new concept of breaking and formation of bonds.

(b) *A molecular picture of junctions*

We give here a molecular picture of intercellular junctions, taking into account some experimental evidence of these junctions swelling due to stimuli or inflammation. Setting aside the question of transendothelial transport of serum albumin, it will be helpful to study those substances of smaller molecular size, which actually pass through junctions.

In the intercellular cleft, different types of junctional complexes are observed with large variations in the intercellular spacing. In order to predict membrane deformation on molecular-level, long-range membrane interaction, simplified models have been put forward. Let us here consider Weinbaum's model (Weinbaum, 1979) of membrane interactions in a continuum context.

This theory includes the mechanical and molecular-level forces under the heterogeneous internal structure of the membrane. The molecular-level forces act primarily between the integral proteins in the same and opposing membrane, and are of a specialized nature depending on their biochemical configuration. One manifestation of this difference lies in the distributions of negative surface charge associated with the carboxyl groups of the sialic acid side chains attached to the exterior surface of the integral proteins. Under the influence of random thermal motion, integral proteins in the same membrane will either be randomly dispersed or will form linear arrays or hexagonal clusters, depending on the balance of electrostatic and van der Waals forces. The latter always produce an attraction between identical particles.

The equilibrium configuration of two adjacent membranes results from the balance of three primary forces: (i) membrane bending stress; (ii) a van der Waals interaction pressure; (iii) electric disjoining pressure arising from the negative charge on the exterior surface of each membrane. Like proteins in opposing membranes will become coupled when the particle arrays in a given membrane are sufficiently large for the van der Waals attraction between the arrays to overcome their lateral Brownian diffusion.

(c) *Homogeneous diffusion theory*

Let us consider the effect of mechanical disturbances on permeability in the homogeneous picture of protoplasm and intercellular junctions (Oka, 1976, 1979). If the van der Waals bond is specified by the mutual potential energy barrier E, the probability p with which the bond is broken is given by

$$p = \exp(-E/RT) \tag{8.12}$$

This means that a fraction of the bonds is always broken due to thermal motion even in a natural, undisturbed state.

Let the number of bonds in the undisturbed state be denoted by N_0, and the corresponding activation energy and diffusion coefficient by E_0 and D_0, respectively. Then we have

$$D_0 = A \exp(-E_0/RT) \tag{8.13}$$

Let the increase in the number of broken bonds under a given mechanical disturbance be denoted by ΔN_b, and the corresponding decrease in the activation energy and the increase in the diffusion coefficient be denoted by ΔE and ΔD, respectively. From the relationship:

$$D_0 + \Delta D = A \exp[-(E_0 - \Delta E)/RT] \tag{8.14}$$

and Eq. (8.13) we have

$$\Delta D = D_0 \frac{\Delta E}{RT} \tag{8.15}$$

where $E/RT \ll 1$ has been taken into account.

Let the increase in the uptake of albumin due to mechanical disturbance be denoted by ΔM. Since the uptake is proportional to the diffusion coefficient, we have $\Delta M \propto \Delta D$, or

$$\Delta M \propto D_0 \frac{\Delta E}{RT} \propto \Delta E \tag{8.16}$$

It is reasonable to expect that the more the bonds are broken down, the more the activation energy decreases,

$$\Delta E \propto \Delta N_b \tag{8.17}$$

The above relation is supported by the statistical theory of zero-

8.8 Vascular permeability to proteins

dimensional gel filtration (Rodbard & Chrambach, 1970). Thus, we have the important result:

$$\Delta M = a\Delta N_b \tag{8.18}$$

where a is a constant. We can conclude that the excess uptake is proportional to the excess number of broken bonds.

(d) Effects of mechanical disturbances
(i) Wall shear stress

The effect of steady wall shear stress τ on the uptake of serum albumin across the endothelial surface, studied by Carew, and Nerem et al., was described in Sect. 8.6. Carew showed that in the shear stress range 100 to 450 dyn cm^{-2}

$$M = c_0 + c_1\tau^2 \tag{8.19}$$

where c_0 and c_1 are positive constants. On the other hand, Nerem et al. showed a slight shear dependence in the shear stress range 10 to 100 dyn cm^{-2}

$$M = c\tau^{0.38} \tag{8.20}$$

where c is a positive constant. The two relationships mentioned above are not contradictory, but they are complementary, because their shear stress ranges are entirely different. Their results can be unified as in Fig. 88. The curve shows an inflection point at the shear stress near 100 dyn cm^{-2}.

If we consider Eq. (8.18), the curve in Fig. 88 can be interpreted as the plot of the excess number of broken bonds against the shear

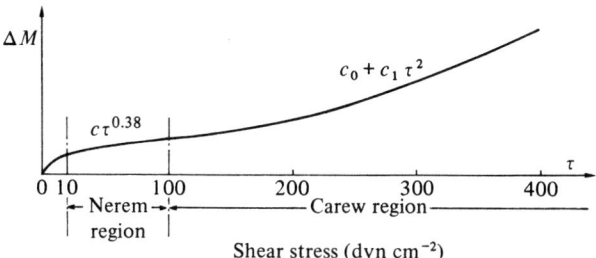

Fig. 88. Surface concentration of albumin in a wide range of shear stress. (From Oka, 1979.)

stress. In order to interpret the above curve theoretically, let us compare it with the distribution curve, $p(\tau)$, of the tensile strength of any material. The total number of broken specimens, $P(\tau)$, for the tensile strength τ is given by

$$P(\tau) = \int_0^\tau p(\tau)\,d\tau \qquad (8.21)$$

Then, if the distribution curve has a maximum at a certain tensile strength τ_m, the integral distribution curve has an inflection point at the same strength, since $d^2P/d\tau^2 = dp/d\tau = 0$ at $\tau = \tau_m$. Consequently, the $\Delta M - \tau$ curve can be understood to correspond to the integral distribution curve $P(\tau)$. The ordinate can also be regarded as representing ΔN_b, the increase in the number of broken bonds. It should be noted that the break-down of bonds in the presence of sinusoidally oscillating flow corresponds to fatigue in solid materials.

(ii) Stretch

As is shown in Fig. 83, the albumin uptake into the wall increases rapidly with increase in the stretch ratio λ. It is clear that stretching increases the mutual potential energy of the van der Waals bond by increasing the mutual distance. Let the depth of the potential energy valley and the increase in the potential energy caused by the stretch ratio λ be denoted by E_0 and ΔE, respectively (Fig. 89).

Fig. 89. Lowering of potential energy barrier.

8.8 Vascular permeability to proteins

The probability that the bond is broken down by thermal motion in the unstretched state is given by

$$p = \exp(-E_0/RT) \tag{8.22}$$

and hence we have the number of broken bonds

$$N_b = N_0 \exp(-E_0/RT) \tag{8.23}$$

where N_0 is a constant. From Eqs. (8.18) and (8.23) we have

$$\Delta M = aN_b \frac{\Delta E}{RT} \tag{8.24}$$

The decrease ΔE is certainly related to the stretch ratio λ. If the protoplasm or the junction can be regarded as a homogeneous continuum, then ΔE is proportional to the strain energy density function W. In the theory of large deformation, W for one-dimensional stretch is given by

$$W = \text{const}\,(\lambda^2 - 1)^2 \tag{8.25}$$

Consequently, we have for the excess uptake ΔM:

$$\Delta M = \text{const}\,(\lambda^2 - 1)^2 \tag{8.26}$$

In order to test the above prediction, the excess uptake ΔM from Fig. 83 was replotted against $(\lambda^2 - 1)^2$. Figure 90 shows the result.

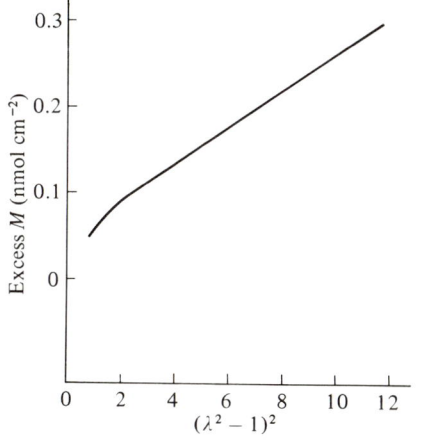

Fig. 90. Excess albumin uptake vs. $(\lambda^2 - 1)^2$. (From Oka, 1979.)

The ratio of ΔM to $(\lambda^2 - 1)^2$ is constant for large values of λ. Another linear portion appears near the ordinate. This can be interpreted as follows: for small values of elongation $\gamma = \lambda - 1$, W is, of course, proportional to γ^2, which is approximately equal to $\frac{1}{4}(\lambda^2 - 1)^2$.

(iii) Wholebody vibration

As described in Sect. 8.6, wholebody vibration data have on average double or more the wall uptake compared with non-vibration data. According to our molecular picture, the increase in the number of broken bonds due to vibration can be understood if we consider the viscoelasticity of the system. Vibration, of course, causes energy loss, i.e. mechanical energy is transformed into heat, which in turn causes the breakdown of bonds. Thus, we can conclude that albumin uptake is enhanced by vibration.

The mechanism of the wholebody vibration effect on albumin uptake will not be simple, since wholebody vibration may not only alter the flow in arteries and wall shear stress; it may also stimulate the nervous system to produce vasoactive substances.

(e) *Vesicle diffusion theory*

The van der Waals and electrical double layer forces may play an important role when biological membranes approach one another. Then, the boundary plasmalemma will affect the passage of a free vesicle through an endothelial cell. Weinbaum (1979) developed a continuum theory for vesicle diffusion based on the interaction of a vesicle with the boundary plasmalemmas. The theory includes the hydrodynamic resistance which the vesicle experiences in squeezing out the water from the intervening fluid gap and the van der Waals force interaction with the boundary plasmalemma. Electrical double layer forces are thought to be much weaker than hydrodynamic and electrodynamic forces, since the exterior surface of the vesicle and the cytoplasmic surface of the plasmalemma do not have significant charge.

They proposed a governing steady-state diffusion equation

$$\frac{d}{dx}(cu) = \frac{d}{dx}\left(D(x)\frac{dc}{dx}\right) \tag{8.27}$$

where the x-axis is taken to be perpendicular to the boundary

8.8 Vascular permeability to proteins

plasmalemma, u is the convective velocity of the vesicle due to the van der Waals forces, c is the concentration of free vesicles, and $D(x)$ is a spatially dependent diffusion coefficient that describes the fluid resistance to a spherical particle moving perpendicularly to two plane parallel boundaries. In the previous diffusion model, $D(x)$ was treated as constant, and long-range electrodynamic interactions were neglected. The expression for u can be obtained by calculating the balance of forces on a vesicle in which the sum of van der Waals, convection gradient and hydrodynamic resistance forces is set equal to zero as follows:

$$0 = F - 6\pi a \mu \lambda u \qquad (8.28)$$

where F is the van der Waals interaction force, a is the vesicle radius, u is the velocity of intervening fluid, and λ is the spatially varying hydrodynamic resistance coefficient. In the above, an approximate expression for λ is assumed in which the fluid resistance increases as the gap width approaches zero. Weinbaum obtained an approximate expression for F by summing the interaction between plasmalemma membranes and all the surface elements comprising the vesicle.

The solution obtained from Eq. (8.28) showed how the vesicle velocity dramatically increases as the plasmalemma is approached. Approximate solutions to Eq. (8.28) were put forward for the free vesicle concentration profiles of vesicles released at the luminal plasmalemma. The curious feature of these solutions is the great influence of the van der Waals force on the concentration profiles of the free vesicles in the cell interior.

The kinetics of vesicle attachment or detachment is affected by the diffusion in the cell interior, and by a permeability coefficient of the average vesicular transport across the endothelial cell layer. If c_p and $c(0)$ are the macromolecule concentrations at the luminal and interstitial surfaces of the endothelial cell, the steady-state permeability coefficient, P, is given by

$$P = J/(c_p - c(0)) \qquad (8.29)$$

where $J = \phi_R V(c_p - c(0))$ is the net macromolecule flux from the lumen to the tissue sides, ϕ_R being the vesicle number flux $\text{cm}^{-2}\,\text{s}^{-1}$, and V being the available filling volume in the vesicle interior.

The approximate expression for P was expected as:

$$P = \frac{NVk\phi_R}{2}\frac{1}{\phi}\frac{1}{1+Y} \qquad Y = \frac{N_f l^2 k}{2D_0} \qquad (8.30)$$

where N is the total number of free and attached vesicles/cm², ϕ_R/ϕ is the probability that a vesicle released at the luminal membrane crosses the cell, N_f a dimensionless free vesicle density/cm² of endothelial surface, k is the rate of rupture of the vesicle neck and the resealing of the vesicle membrane, l is the diffusion distance, and D_0 is the standard diffusion coefficient. Both ϕ_R/ϕ and N_f are functions of the effective van der Waals range ε for a given cell and vesicle geometry. It can be seen that when $Y \ll 1$, the permeability is controlled by the probability ϕ_R/ϕ that the vesicle will cross the cell and thus is sensitive to ε. When $Y \gg 1$ the increase in the free vesicle density function N_f with decreasing ε just cancels out the increase in probability that vesicle will cross the cell, with the result that the steady-state permeability is independent of ε.

8.9 Stresses in the arterial wall as a cause of permeability

The permeability of arteries is affected not only by the blood flow in the arteries, but also by the stretch of the arterial walls. We now consider the relation between the stresses in the arterial walls and their permeability.

(a) Hypertension and permeability

Hypertension and atherosclerosis are closely associated; many factors are involved in both diseases, and their interrelation is very complicated. Here we limit ourselves to the direct effect of hypertension on the permeability of arterial walls.

As stated in Chapter 6, the circumferential tension in a blood vessel wall is generally given by

$$T_c = p_1 r_1 - p_2 r_2 \qquad (8.31)$$

where p_1 and p_2 are, respectively, the internal and external pressures, and r_1 and r_2 are the inner and outer radii of the vessel under the pressures p_1 and p_2. When the tension T_c is calculated under normal blood pressure from Eq. (8.31), employing values for r_1 and r_2 from existing data, T_c is negative in all blood vessels other than the

8.9 Arterial wall stresses: cause of permeability

aorta and vena cava; most blood vessels are in a state of compression. In this case, our molecular picture suggests that the uptake of substances into blood vessel walls is generally prevented. As blood pressure increases, T_c changes from negative to positive, suggesting that permeability is increased by hypertension.

The permeability of an arterial wall depends most on the circumferential stress τ_θ at the endothelium. If we assume, for simplicity, that the arterial wall is homogeneous and obeys Hooke's law, then τ_θ at the endothelium can be obtained by putting $r = r_1$ in Eq. (6.15). If we introduce the parameters $k = p_1/p_2$ and $s = r_2/r_1$, then τ_θ can be rewritten as

$$\tau_\theta = p_2[k(1 + s^2) - 2s^2]/(s^2 - 1) \tag{8.32}$$

Let us consider the sk-plane, k being the ordinate. The stress τ_θ becomes zero on the curve

$$k = 2s^2/(1 + s^2) \tag{8.33}$$

The upper region corresponds to $\tau_\theta > 0$ and the lower to $\tau_\theta < 0$. Our molecular picture suggests that the blood vessel wall is protected from atherosclerosis in the region $\tau_\theta < 0$, while atherosclerosis may be expected in the region $\tau_\theta > 0$.

Johshita et al. (1978) developed a method of local control of intravascular pressure, and applied it to various arteries of a rabbit. The arterial lesion did not directly correlate with intravascular pressure, but was closely related to change in the circumferential tension, T_c. When the intra-arterial pressure was controlled in various arteries from human autopsies, it was found that the hypertensive arterial lesion was apt to develop in the part (for example, cerebral arteries) where it was easy to induce positive value of T_c.

(b) Stress concentration in arterial branching

As already mentioned, atherosclerotic plaques tend to develop at arterial branchings. Niimi (1979) detected high stress concentration in the intimal surface of the branch, and suggested that this is an important localizing factor in atherosclerosis.

The arterial wall may be stretched or deformed at branchings more easily than elsewhere because there is no elastic medium to moderate blood pressure and axial tetherings. In a simple model of branching (an infinitely long cylindrical shell of homogeneous, isotropic Hookean wall with a circular hole for branching) exists, in the intimal surface of the branch, a high stress concentration which depends on the branching specification. Thus one can view arterial branches as suffering from local hypertension since their walls are subjected to high tension with large stress pulsation.

The predicted high stress concentration in the intimal surface may increase the permeability of the arterial wall. The conclusion is that high stress concentration in arterial branchings is responsible for the development of atherosclerosis at this point. This is supported by the common knowledge that chronic hypertension may accelerate the progress of atherosclerosis.

(c) *Regional permeability in an aneurysmal dilation*

Aneurysmal dilations are often observed in the arterial system. Niimi & Oka (1979) studied the stress distribution in an

Fig. 91. Stress distribution in an aneurysmal dilation. T_L: longitudinal tension; p: transmural pressure. (From Niimi & Oka, 1979.)

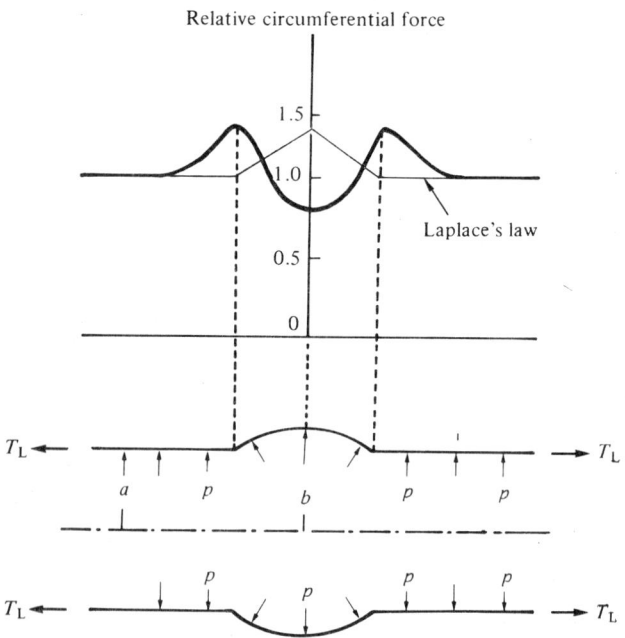

aneurysmal dilation using an axisymmetric model, which is composed of a straight portion of radius a, and the aneurysmal portion of radius b (Fig. 91). They assumed that the arterial wall is homogeneous, isotropic and Hookean, and that the model is subjected to the axial tethering force and uniform pressure, and applied the *thin shell theory* developed in solid mechanics to the two portions, matching the deflection, the angle of deflection, the resultant forces and moments at the junction of the two portions. They found that the relative circumferential force is largest at the ends of the aneurysmal dilation, i.e. at the junction of the aneurysmal and the straight portions, and is smallest at the point of largest dilation. Their findings cannot be predicted by Laplace's law, suggesting that aneurysm may be caused by the highly concentrated stress and deformation at the ends of the small dilations in arterioles.

8.10 Interaction of blood flow and arterial endothelium

It is important in pathophysiology to know how the arterial wall responds to changes in pressure and other stresses, and especially to know the long-term response to various stresses caused by the interaction of blood flow and arterial endothelium.

In normal blood vessels, the shear stress caused by blood flow is thought to be much smaller than the critical shear stress produced by Fry. This is backed by recent studies of the interaction of white cells with the endothelium, in which white cells are often seen sticking to the endothelium or rolling slowly along it, while the red cells and plasma flow around them.

Yu & Goldsmith (1973) carried out some experimental studies of blood cell behavior in vortices near a spherical obstruction. A 650 μm diameter polystyrene sphere was fused onto the wall of a 1000 μm diameter glass tube with a dilute red cell suspension flowing downward at a mean flow rate of 3.1 cm s^{-1}. Flow velocities here were too large to permit tracking of particles in the microtube, but the paths of the particles in and close to the vortex region were obtained by taking high-speed cine films. They found that flow separation occurs distal to the obstruction and a vortex forms through which the cells move in spiral orbits. Fig. 92 shows the spiral orbits followed by red cells in the vortex downstream of the spherical obstruction.

By high-speed filming of the flow around the white cell sticking to the endothelium, the flow field may be determined. Then the force of interaction of the white cell and the endothelium can be calculated either theoretically or according to data from experiments with models. In fact, Schmid-Schönbein, Fung & Zweifach (1975) found that the normal stress of interaction between the white cell

Fig. 92. Red cell paths downstream of a spherical obstacle. (From Yu & Goldsmith, 1973.)

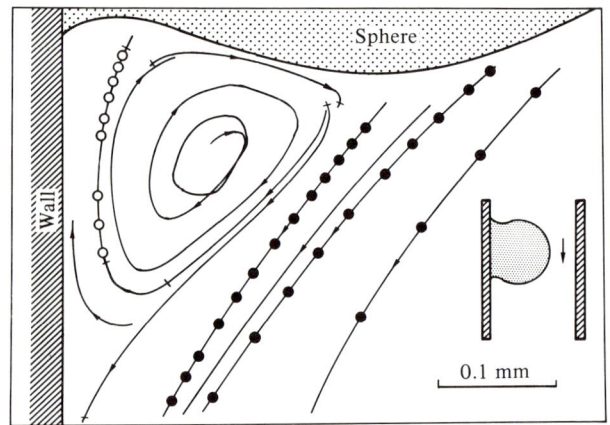

Fig. 93. Separation region and flow velocity downstream of a micro-obstacle. (From Niimi & Yamakawa, 1980.)

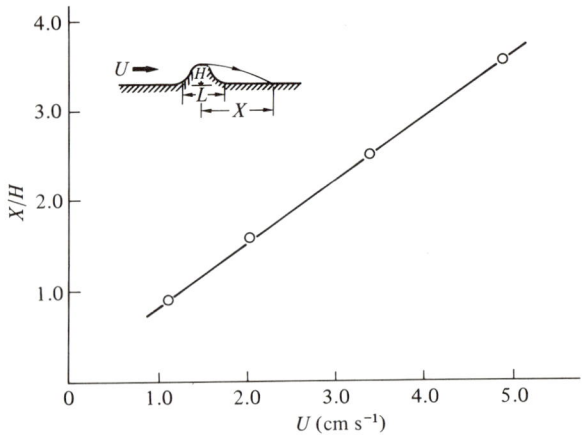

8.10 Blood flow and arterial endothelium

and endothelium has a maximum value of the same order of magnitude as the shear stress.

There is much morphological evidence of wavy ultrastructures at the intima. The ultrastructure may play a role in the fine structure of blood flow, which in turn affects the interaction of the blood and endothelium. Recently, Niimi & Yamakawa (1980) determined the fine structure of blood flow around a plaque-like structure of wall, using data from experiments with models. They found that flow separation occurs distal to the micro-obstacle fused on the wall and that a vortex forms through which the red cells oscillate. Figure 93 shows the length of vortices distal to the obstacle against the flow velocity proximal to the micro-obstacle with the height of 0.5 mm. Note the quasi-steady vortex extremely near the micro-obstacle which represents an atherosclerotic plaque.

In the formation of thrombosis, the collision of platelets with the wall may play an important role. The frequency is expected to be higher in regions where the particles are carried by radially directed streamlines toward the wall, immediately upstream of the reattachment points; it will be relatively low near the separation point, where the particles are carried away from the wall (Yu & Goldsmith, 1973). When the endothelium is damaged and the underlying collagen fibers are exposed to the circulating blood, the collision efficiency becomes appreciable because of the platelets high affinity for collagen.

Supplement to Sect. 8.4 (added in proof)

As is well known, electric double layers exist at the boundaries between plasma and blood cells and between plasma and the endothelial cell membranes. Then, the *intermembrane potential* will play an important role in the mechanism of thrombus formation; if the collision of platelets with the wall is suppressed under the existence of the potential, thrombus formation will not take place, but if platelets in turbulent flow are supplied with kinetic energy enough to overcome the barrier of the potential, thrombus formation may actually take place.

9

Prospects for cardiovascular hemorheology in the future

As early as 1951 Copley introduced the term 'hemorheology' for the rheology of blood and blood vessels. In 1962 the first issue of the international journal *Biorheology* was published through his efforts. Following his proposal, the First International Conference on Hemorheology was held in Reykjavik in 1966. At that time the International Society of Hemorheology was organized, and it was decided that future international conferences should take place every three years. The Second International Conference on Hemorheology took place in Heidelberg, where it was decided that future conferences should include all fields of rheology in biological systems. Thus the Society's name was changed to the International Society of Biorheology. Yet the most presentations at each International Congress of Biorheology were in the field of hemorheology; and the same happened with the journal *Biorheology*. Investigation of hemorheology in many countries is increasing.

There is a very good reason why hemorheology has grown so rapidly. Blood circulation is, of course, necessary for life, and hence circulatory disorders are the most fatal. To understand blood circulation and circulatory disorders, hemorheological studies are essential; but the knowledge of hemorheology was very rudimentary until the middle of this century. In the 1950s and 1960s some rheologists turned to the study of hemorheology, and also some medical scientists became particularly interested in clinical hemotheology.

Blood circulation is a medical field, whereas rheology is a field of science which is closely related to physics, chemistry, biology and technology. Hemorheology has two sides: the main purpose is medical, while the methodology comes from science and technology. Therefore, high-level studies of hemorheology can only be carried out with the cooperation of investigators from both fields. This feature can easily be seen in presentations at the International Conference of Hemorheology or Biorheology and the papers in *Biorheology*. Of course, model experiments and theoretical studies are emphasized by engineers and physicists. It is expected that new hemorheological concepts and techniques will enable clinical hemorheology to expand markedly.

In many natural sciences, it is a common feature of scientific research that a problem is studied deeply within a narrow area. In the case of a multidisciplinary research as hemorheology, both specialization and synthesis play an important role. Otherwise no real progress in hemorheology can occur. Atherogenesis is a good example of multidisciplinary approach, in which hemorheological studies play an important role.

There is a general trend that scientific research starts from macroscopic phenomena and then proceeds to the microscopic basis underlying these phenomena. In this respect rheology is no exception, and a new field, '*microrheology*', has already developed. The same has happened with hemorheology. The deformability and special rheological behavior of red cells have now become very important in '*microhemorheology*'.

It is very difficult to predict the future of hemorheology from its present course. But we can expect the following:

(i) Cooperation among clinicians, scientists and engineers in various areas will become increasingly active.

(ii) Quantitative observations will be more accurate with new highly sophisticated methods and technical procedures.

(iii) A number of measuring instruments will be developed based on new physical and chemical principles which have not previously been applied to hemorheology.

(iv) Highly sophisticated studies by scientists and engineers may solve some medical problems which still baffle clinicians.

(v) Although hemorheology has the two different sides, any separation of these will have an adverse effect.

(vi) Very few chemists are interested in hemorheology at present. Knowledge of surface chemistry and surface rheology will greatly aid the study of the interface between blood and blood vessels.

(vii) Problems which have scarcely been studied, such as the flow of tissue fluid among the cells, will prove to be of great interest.

(viii) One of the most important problems in cadiovascular hemorheology concerns with the interaction of blood and blood vessels at their interface. Microscopic studies involving electric double layers with zeta potentials will play a role of increasing importance. Their significance particularly in microcirculation is obvious.

Readers of this book will find many experimental results as well as theories which need further detailed investigation. This is partly due to the fact that hemorheology is a relatively new subject. This small book will help readers to develop their studies of cardiovascular hemorheology.

References

Chapter 1

Green, H. D. (1944). Circulation: physical principles. In *Medical Physics*, ed. O. Glasser, vol. 1, p. 208, Year Book Medical Publishers, Chicago.

Chapter 2

Blasius, H. (1913). Das Ähnlichkeitsgesetz der Reibungsvorgängen in Flüssigkeiten. *Forschg. Arb. Ing.-Wes.*, no. 131, Berlin.

Einstein, A. (1906). Eine neue Bestimmung der Moleküldimensionen. *Ann. Physik* **19**, 289.

Eirich, F. R., Bunzl, M. & Margaretta, H. (1936). Untersuchungen über die Viskosität von Suspensionen und Lösungen 4. Über die Viskosität von Kugel-suspensionen. *Kolloid-Z.* **74**, 276.

Goldsmith, H. L. & Mason, S. G. (1975). Some model experiments in hemodynamics–V: microrheological techniques. *Biorheology* **12**, 181.

Taylor, G. I. (1932). The viscosity of a fluid containing small drops of another fluid. *Proc. Roy. Soc.* **138A**, 41.

Whitmore, R. L. (1968). *Rheology of the Circulation*, p. 113. Pergamon Press, Oxford.

Chapter 3

Barbee, J. H. & Cokelet, G. R. (1971). The Fahraeus effect. *Microvasc. Res.* **3**, 6.

Bate, H. (1977). Blood viscosity at different shear rates in capillary tubes. *Biorheology* **14**, 267.

Bayliss, L. E. (1952). Rheology of blood and lymph. In *Deformation and Flow in Biological Systems*, ed. A. Frey-Wyssling. North-Holland, Amsterdam.

Bayliss, L. E. (1959). The axial drift of red cells when blood flows in a narrow tube. *J. Physiol.* **149**, 593.

Casson, N. (1959). A flow equation for pigment–oil suspensions of the printing ink type. In *Rheology of Disperse Systems*, ed. C. C. Mill, p. 84. Pergamon Press, Oxford.

Charm, S. E. & Kurland, G. S. (1972). Blood rheology. In *Cardiovascular Fluid Dynamics*, ed. D. H. Bergel. Academic Press, London.

Charm, S. E., Kurland, G. S. & Brown, S. L. (1968). The influence of radial distribution and marginal plasma layer on the flow of red cell suspensions. *Biorheology* **5**, 15.

Chien, S. (1975). Biophysical behavior of red cells in suspensions. In *The Red Blood Cell*, 2nd edn., ed. D. MacN. Surgenor, vol. 2, p. 1031. Academic Press, New York.

Chien, S., Usami, S., Taylor, H., Leniberg, J. S. & Gregersen, M. (1966). The effect of hematocrit and plasma protein on human blood rheology at low shear rates. *J. Appl. Physiol.* **21**, 81.

Copley, A. L. (1958). Adherence and viscosity of blood contacting foreign surfaces, and the plasmatic zone in blood circulation. *Nature* **181**, 551.

Copley, A. L. (1979). Certain aspects of hemorheology in a near-zero gravity environment. *Biorheology* **16**, 37.

Copley, A. L., King, R. G., Chien, S., Usami, S., Skalak, K. & Huang, C. R. (1975). Microscopic observations of viscoelasticity of human blood in steady and oscillatory shear. *Biorheology* **12**, 257.

Copley, A. L., Luchini, B. N. & Whelan, E. W. (1967). On the role of fibrinogen–fibrin complexes in flow properties and suspension stability of blood systems. *Biorheology* **4**, 87.

Copley, A. L. & Scott Blair, G. W. (1961). Comparative observations on adherence and consistency of various blood systems in living and artificial capillaries. *Rheol. Acta* **1**, 170; 665.

Copley, A. L., Scott Blair, G. W., Glover, F. A. & Thorley, R. S. (1960). Capillary flow and wall adherence of bovine blood, plasma and serum in contact with glass and fibrin surfaces. *Kolloid-Z.* **168**, 101.

Dintenfass, L. (1975). Internal viscosity of the red cell: problems associated with definition of plasma viscosity and effective volume of red cells in the blood viscosity equation. *Biorheology* **12**, 253.

Dintenfass, L. (1979). Aggregation of red cells and blood viscosity under near-zero gravity. *Biorheology* **16**, 29.

Dix, F. S. & Scott Blair, G. W. (1940). On the flow of suspensions through narrow tubes. *J. Appl. Phys.* **11**, 574.

Fahraeus, R. (1929). The suspension stability of blood. *Physiol. Rev.* **9**, 241.

Fahraeus, R. & Lindqvist, T. (1931a). The viscosity of blood in narrow capillary tubes. *Amer. J. Physiol.* **76**, 562.

Fahraeus, R. & Lindqvist, T. (1931b). Human blood. *Amer. J. Physiol.* **96**, 562.

Fukada, E. & Kaibara, M. (1973). The dynamic rigidity of fibrin gels. *Biorheology* **10**, 129.

Gaehtgens, P., Albrecht, K. H. & Kreutz, F. (1978a). Fahraeus effect and cell screening during tube flow of human blood. I. Effect of variation of flow rate. *Biorheology* **15**, 147.

Gaehtgens, P., Kreutz, F. & Albrecht, K. H. (1978b). Fahraeus effect and cell screening during tube flow of human blood. II. Effect of dextran-induced cell aggregation. *Biorheology* **15**, 155.

Goldsmith, H. L. & Mason, S. G. (1965). Further comments on the radial migration of spheres in Poiseuille flow. *Biorheology* **3**, 33.

Gordon, W. (1970). Modified marginal zone theory of blood flow through a rigid tube. *Biorheology* **7**, 125.

Hartert, H. (1960). Thrombelastography: physical and physiological aspects. In *Flow Properties of Blood and Other Biological Systems*, ed. A. L. Copley & G. Stainsby, p. 186. Pergamon Press, Oxford.

Haynes, R. H. (1960). Physical basis of the dependence of blood viscosity on tubes radius. *Amer. J. Physiol.* **198**, 1193.

Haynes, R. H. & Burton, A. C. (1959). Role of the non-Newtonian behavior of blood in hemodynamics. *Amer. J. Physiol.* **197**, 943.

Healy, J. C. & Joly, M. (1975). Rheological behavior of blood in transient flow. *Biorheology* **12**, 335.

Hess, W. R. (1912). Der Strömungswiederstand des Blutes gegenüber kleinen Druckwerten. *Arch. Physiol.* p. 197.

Heuser, G. (1978). Secondary effects in cone and plate viscometers. *Biorheology* **15**, 311.

Huang, C. R., Siskovic, N., Robertson, R. W., Fabisiak, W., Smitherberg, E. H. & Copley, A. L. (1975). Quantitative characterization of thixotropy of whole human blood. *Biorheology* **12**, 279.

Inouye, A., Kamino, K., Ogawa, M. & Uyesaka, N. (1976). Pressure–flow relation of erythrocyte suspension in perfusion of bullfrog's hind limb and marginal zone theory. *Biorheology* **13**, 251.

Jan, K. (1979). Red cell interactions in macromolecular suspension. *Biorheology* **16**, 137.

Kaibara, M. & Fukada, E. (1969). Non-Newtonian viscosity and dynamic viscoelasticity of blood during clotting. *Biorheology* **6**, 73.

Kaibara, M. & Fukada, E. (1971). The influence of the concentration of thrombin on the dynamic viscoelasticity of clotting blood and fibrinogen–thrombin systems. Biorheology **8**, 139.

Kimzey, S. L., (1979). A review of hematology studies associated with space flight. *Biorheology* **16**, 13.

King, R. G. & Copley, A. L. (1975). Some new accessories to the Weissenberg Rheogoniometer; an exhibit. *Biorheology* **12**, 355.

Knox, R. J., Nordt, F. J., Seaman, G. V. F. & Brooks D. E. (1977). Rheology of erythrocyte suspensions: dextran-mediated aggregation of deformable and nondeformable erythrocytes. *Biorheology* **14**, 75.

Koyama, K., Kitahara, R., Kanamaru, K. & Wada, E. (1967). Effect of wall surface on capillary flow. *Zairyo* **16**, 525 (in Japanese).

Koyama, K., Oki, N., Kanamaru, K. & Wada, E. (1970). Effect of wall surface on capillary flow. *Rep. Prog. Polymer Phys. Japan* **13**, 95.

Koyama, K., Ooi, E., Wada, E. & Kanamaru, K. (1971). Effect of wall surface on capillary flow. III. Effect of fibrin coating. *Rep. Prog. Polymer Phys. Japan* **14**, 635.

Maude, A. D. & Whitmore, R. L. (1958). Theory of the flow of blood in narrow tubes. *J. Appl. Physiol.* **12**, 105.

Merrill, E. W., Gilliland, E. R., Cokelet, G. R., Shin, H., Britten, A. & Wells, R. E. (1963). Rheology of human blood – effects of temperature and hematocrit level. *Biophys. J.* **3**, 199.

Merrill, E. W., Margetts, W. G., Cokelet, G. R. & Gilliland, E. R. (1965). The Casson equation and rheology of blood near zero shear. *Symposium of Biorheology*, ed. A. L. Copley, p. 135.

Müller, A. (1942). Abhandlungen zur Mechanik der Flüssigkeiten mit besonderer Berücksichtigung der Hämodynamik: Strömen in Röhren: Strömung von Suspensionen in Röhrean. *Arch. Kreislaufforsch.* **8**, 245.

Murata, T. (1976). Theory of non-Newtonian viscosity of blood at low shear rate–effect of rouleaux. *Biorheology* **13**, 287.

Oka, S. (1965). Theoretical considerations on the flow of blood through a capillary. In *Symposium on Biorheology*, ed. A. L. Copley, p. 89. Wiley Interscience, New York.

Oka, S. (1967). Rheology of blood. *Kobunshi* **16**, 742 (in Japanese).

Oka, S. (1968). Theoretical approach to the effect of wall surface condition in hemorheology. In *Hemorheology*, ed. A. L. Copley, p. 55. Pergamon Press, Oxford.

Oka, S. (1971). An approach to a unified theory of the flow behavior of time-independent non-Newtonian suspensions. *Japan. J. Appl. Phys.* **10**, 287.

Ossoff, R. & Charm, S. E. (1974). Blood viscosity reduction in negative charged capillary tubes. *Biorheology* **11**, 293.

Overholser, K. A., Itin, J. P., Brown D. R. & Harris, T. R. (1975). The effect of heparin on the viscoelasticity of whole blood clots. *Biorheology* **12**, 309.

Palmer, A. A. & Betts, W. H. (1975). The axial drift of fresh and acetaldehyde hardened erythrocytes in 25 μm capillary slits of various lengths. *Biorheology* **12**, 283.

Palmer, A. A. & Jedrzejczyk, H. J. (1975). The influence of rouleaux on the resistance to flow through capillary channels at various shear rates. *Biorheology* **12**, 265.

Phillips, W. M. & Deutsch, S. (1975). Toward a constitutive equation for blood. *Biorheology* **12**, 383.

Poiseuille, J. L. M. (1836). *Ann. des Sciences Naturelles, Sér.* 2, *Zool.* **5**, 111.

Puccini, C., Stasiw, D. M. & Cerny, L. C. (1977). The erythrocyte sedimentation curve: a semi-empirical approach. *Biorheology* **14**, 43.

Sacks, A. H., Little, H. L. & Kirk, K. W. (1977). Quantification of the degree of red cell aggregation using a Wells–Brookfield rheoscope. *Biorheology* **14**, 99.

Saville, D. A. (1979). Flow processes in a micro-gravity environment. *Biorheology* **16**, 23.

Schmid-Schönbein, H. (1977). Microrheology of erythrocytes and thrombocytes, blood viscosity and the distribution of blood flow in the microcirculation. In *Microcirculation*, ed. H. Meessen, p. 305. Springer-Verlag, Berlin.

Scott Blair, G. W. (1958). The importance of sigma phenomena in the flow of blood. *Rheol. Acta* **1**, 123.

Scott Blair, G. W. (1959). An equation for the flow of blood, plasma and serum through glass capillaries. *Nature* **183**, 613.

References

Scott Blair, G. W. (1974). *An Introduction to Biorheology*, p. 71. Elsevier Scientific, Amsterdam.

Segré, G. & Silberberg, A. (1962). Behaviour of macroscopic rigid spheres in Poiseuille flow. *J. Fluid Mech.* **14**, 115.

Shiga, T., Maeda, N., Suda, T., Kon, K., Sekiya, M. & Oka, S. (1979). Rheological and kinetic dysfunctions of the cholesterol-loaded, human erythrocytes. *Biorheology* **16**, 363.

Smith, J. R. & Landaw, S. A. (1978). Smokers' polycythemia. *New Engl. J. Medicine* **298**, no. 1.

Snyder, R. S. & Seaman, G. V. F. (1979). Experimentation in space and biorheology. *Biorheology* **16**, 7.

Stein, P. D. & Sabbah, H. N. (1975). Contribution of erythrocytes to turbulent blood flow. *Biorheology* **12**, 293.

Tamamushi, B. (1971). Surface chemical aspects of flow characteristics of blood. In *Theoretical and Clinical Hemorheology*, ed. H. H. Hartert & A. L. Copley, p. 99. Springer-Verlag, Berlin.

Taylor, M. G. (1955). The flow of blood in narrow tubes. II. The axial stream and its formation, as determined by changes in optical density. *Aust. J. Exp. Biol. Med. Sci.* **33**, 1.

Thomas, D. J., Marshall, J., Russel, R. W. R., Wetherley-Mein, G., du Boulay, G. H., Pearson, T. C., Snyder, L. & Zilkha, E. (1977). Effect of hematocrit on cerebral blood-flow in man. *The Lancet*, vol. II, 941.

Thurston, G. B. (1973). Frequency and shear rate dependence of viscoelasticity of human blood. *Biorheology* **10**, 375.

Thurston, G. B. (1979). Rheological parameters for the viscosity, viscoelasticity and thixotropy of blood. *Biorheology* **16**, 149

Toms, B. A. (1949). Some observations on the flow of linear polymer solutions through straight tubes at large Reynolds numbers. *Proceedings of the 1st International Congress on Rheology*, vol. 2, p. 135. North-Holland, Amsterdam.

Usami, S., King, R. G., Chien, S., Skalak, R., Huang, C. R. & Copley, A. L. (1975). Microcinephotographic studies on red cell aggregation in steady and oscillatory shear – a note. *Biorheology* **12**, 323.

Vincent, N. M. & Oliver, D. R. (1977). Blood sedimentation at controlled shear rates. *Biorheology* **14**, 51.

Walburn, F. J. & Schneck, D. J. (1976). A constitutive equation for whole human blood. *Biorheology* **13**, 201.

Wells, R. E., Merrill, E. W. & Gabelnick, H. (1962). Shear-rate dependence of viscosity of blood: interaction of red cells and plasma proteins. *Trans. Soc. Rheol.* **6**, 19.

Whitmore, R. L. (1959). The viscous flow of disperse suspensions in tubes. In *Rheology of Disperse Systems*, ed. C. C. Mill, p. 49. Pergamon Press, Oxford.

Yen, R. T. & Fung, Y. C. (1977). Inversion of Fahraeus effect and effect of mainstream flow on capillary hematocrit. *J. Appl. Physiol.* **42 (4)**, 578.

Chapter 4

Allard, C., Mohandas, N. & Bessis, M. (1978). Red cell deformability changes in hemolytic anemias estimated by diffractometric methods (ektacytometry). In *Red Cell Rheology*, ed. M. Bessis, S. B. Shohet & N. Mohandas, p. 209. Springer-Verlag, Berlin.

Bessis, M. & Mohandas, N. (1975). A diffractometric method for the measurement of cellular deformability. *Blood Cells* **1**, 307.

Blank, M. & Britten, J. S. (1975). Membrane proteins and membrane rheology. *Biorheology* **12**, 271.

Bull, B. S. (1978). The implications of rheology for red cell membrane structure. In *Red Cell Rheology*, ed. M. Bessis, S. B. Shohet & N. Mohandas, p. 427. Springer-Verlag, Berlin.

Bull, B. S., Brailsford, J. D. & Korpman, R. A. (1978). Red cell membrane deformability: an examination of two apparently disparate methods of measurement. In *Red Cell Rheology*, ed. M. Bessis, S. B. Shohet & N. Mohandas, p. 39. Springer-Verlag, Berlin.

Burton, A. C. (1972). The erythrocytes. In *Physiology and Biophysics of the Circulation*, 2nd edn., p. 22, Year Book Medical Publishers, Chicago.

Canham. P. B. (1970). The minimum energy of bending as a possible explanation of the biconcave shape of the human red blood cell. *J. Theor. Biol.* **26**, 61.

Chien, S. (1978a). Principles and techniques for assessing erythrocyte deformability. In *Red Cell Rheology*, ed. M. Bessis, S. B. Shohet & N. Mohandas, p. 71. Springer-Verlag, Berlin.

Chien, S. (1978b). Rheology of sickle cells and erythrocyte content. In *Red Cell Rheology*, ed. M. Bessis, S. B. Shohet & N. Mohandas, p. 279. Springer-Verlag, Berlin.

Chien, S., Dellenback, R. J., Usami, S. Seaman, G. V. F. & Gregersen, M. I. (1968). Centrifugal packing of suspensions of erythrocytes hardened with acetaldehyde. *Proc. Soc. Exp. Biol. Med.* **127**, 982.

Danielli, J. F. & Davson, H. (1935). A contribution to the theory of permeability of thin films. *J. Cell Comp. Physiol.* **5**, 495.

Ehrly, A. M. (1975). Beeinflussung der Verformbarkeit der Erythrozyten durch Pentoxifyllin. *Med. Welt* **26**, Heft 51, 2300.

Feo, C. & Mohandas, N. (1978). Role of ATP depletion on red cell shape and deformability. In *Red Cell Rheology*, ed. M. Bessis, S. B. Shohet & N. Mohandas, p. 153. Springer-Verlag, Berlin.

Fischer, T. & Schmid-Schönbein, H. (1978). Tank tread motion of red cell membranes in viscometric flow: behavior of intracellular and extracellular markers. In *Red Cell Rheology*, ed. M. Bessis, S. B. Shohet & N. Mohandas, p. 347. Springer-Verlag, Berlin.

Fung, Y. C. (1977). Red blood cells and their deformability. In *microcirculation*, vol. 1, ed. G. Kaley & B. M. Altura, p. 255. University Park Press, Baltimore.

Hochmuth, R. M., Mohandas, N. & Blackshear, P. L., Jr. (1973). Measurement of the elastic modulus for red cell membrane using a fluid mechanical technique. *Biophys. J.* **13**, 747.

Kumar, R. S. (1976). Rheology of blood. I. Energy absorption by membrane of RBC during flow? *Biorheology* **13**, 235.

References

LaCelle, P. L. (1971). Alteration of membrane deformability in hemolytic anemias. In *The Red Cell Membrane*, ed. R. I. Weed, E. R. Jaffé & P. A. Miescher. Grune and Stratton, New York.

Leblond, P. (1973). The discocyte–echinocyte transformation of the human red cell: deformability characteristics. In *Red Cell Shape*, p. 95. Springer-Verlag, Berlin.

Meiselman, H. J. & Baker, R. F. (1977). Flow behavior of ATP-depleted human erythrocytes. *Biorheology* **14**, 111.

Nakao, M., Nakao, T. & Yamazoe, S. (1960). Adenosine triphosphate and maintenance of shape of the human red cell. *Nature* **187**, 945.

Sabbah, H. N. & Stein, P. D. (1976). Effect of erythrocytic deformability upon turbulent blood flow. *Biorheology* **13**, 309.

Schmid-Schönbein, H., Gosen, J. V., Heinich, L., Klose, H. J. & Volger, E. (1973). A counter-rotating 'rheoscope chamber' for the study of the microrheology of blood cell aggregation by microscopic observation and microphotometry. *Microvasc. Res.* **6**, 366.

Shiga, T., Maeda, N., Suda, T., Kon, K., Sekiya, M. & Oka, S. (1979a). Rheological and kinetic dysfunction of the cholesterol-loaded, human erythrocytes. *Biorheology* **16**, 363.

Shiga, T., Maeda, N., Suda, T., Kon, K. & Sekiya, M. (1979b). The decreased membrane fluidity of in vivo aged, human erythrocytes: spin label study. *Biochim. Biophys. Acta* **553**, 84.

Singer, S. J. (1975). Architecture and topography of biologic membranes. In *Cell Membrane*, ed. G. Weissmann & R. Claiborne, p. 35. HP Publishing Co., New York.

Singer, S. J. & Nicolson, G. L. (1972). The fluid mosaic model of the structure of cell membranes. *Science* **175**, 720.

Weed, R. I., LaCelle, P. I. & Merrill, E. W. (1969). Metabolic dependence of red cell membrane deformability. *J. Clin. Invest.* **48**, 795.

Chapter 5

An, K. & Salathe, E. P. (1976). The effect of variable capillary radius and filtration coefficient on fluid exchange. *Biorheology* **13**, 367.

Apelblat, A., Katchalsky, A. K. & Silberberg, A. (1974). A mathematical analysis of capillary–tissue fluid exchange. *Biorheology* **11**, 1.

Asano, M., Ohkubo, C., Ogawa, S., Miyazaki, K. & Miwa, R. (1975a). Cutaneous microcirculatory responses to insulin administration in the fasted normal rabbit, with special regard to peripheral circulating leukocytes. *Microvasc. Res.* **9**, 64.

Asano, M., Ohkubo, C., Ogawa, S. Miyazaki, K. & Miwa R. (1975b). Cutaneous microcirculatory responses to insulin administration in the fasted and hexamethonium treated rabbit, with special regard to peripheral circulating leukocytes. *Microvasc. Res.* **10**, 180.

Bugliarello, G. & Hsiao, G. C. (1970). A mathematical model of the flow in the axial plasmatic gaps of the smaller vessels. *Biorheology* **7**, 5.

Duda, J. L. & Vrentas, J. S. (1971). Steady flow in the region of closed streamlines in a cylindrical cavity. *J. Fluid Mech.* **45**, 247. Heat transfer in a cylindrical cavity. *J. Fluid Mech.* **45**, 261.

Fung, Y. C. & Sobin, S. S. (1969). Theory of sheet flow in lung alveoli. *J. Appl. Physiol.* **26**, 472.

Isogai, Y. (1976). Hemorheological study on microthrombi in diabetes. *Proceedings of the 18th International Congress on Hematology*, Kyoto, p. 740.

'Krogh, A. (1919). The number and distribution of capillaries in muscles with calculations of the oxygen pressure head necessary for supplying the tissue. *J. Physiol.* **52**, 409.

Landis, E. M. (1927). Micro-injection studies of capillary permeability. II. The relation between capillary pressure and the rate at which fluid passes through the walls of single capillaries. *Amer. J. Physiol.* **82**, 217.

Lee, J. S. (1969). Slow viscous flow in a lung alveoli model. *J. Biomech.* **2**, 187.

Lee, J. S. & Fung, Y. C. (1969). Stokes flow around a circular cylindrical post confined between two parallel plates. *J. Fluid Mech.* **37**, 657.

Lew H. S. & Fung, Y. C. (1969a). The motion of the plasma between the red cells in the bolus flow. *Biorheology* **6**, 109.

Lew, H. S. & Fung, Y. C. (1969b). Flow in an occluded circular cylindrical tube with permeable wall. *ZAMP* **20**, 750.

Lighthill, M. J. (1969). In *Symposium on Circulatory and Respiratory Mass Transport*, ed. G. E. W. Wolstenholme & J. Knight, p. 85. Churchill, London.

Murata, T. (1978). Theoretical analysis of transcapillary fluid exchange: the effect of filtration coefficient and lymph flow on fluid exchange. *Microvasc. Res.* **16**, 237.

Oka, S. (1979). Non-Newtonian blood flow in a capillary with a permeable wall. Festschrift of Harold Wayland Symposium, California Institute of Technology, Pasadena.

Oka, S. & Murata, T. (1970). A theoretical study of the flow of blood in a capillary with permeable wall. The 17th Rheology Symposium, Sapporo, 1969. Zairyo **17**, 300 (in Japanese); *Japan. J. Appl. Phys.* **9**, 345.

Prothero, J. & Burton, A. C. (1962). The physics of blood flow in capillaries. II. The capillary resistance to flow. *Biophys. J.* **2**, 199.

Shiga, T., Maeda, N., Suda, T., Kon, K., Sekiya, M. & Oka, S. (1979). Biological and kinetic dysfunctions of the cholesterol loaded human erythrocytes. *Biorheology* **16**, 363.

Skalak, R., Chen, P. H. & Chien, S. (1972). Effect of hematocrit and rouleaux on apparent viscosity in capillaries. *Biorheology* **9**, 67.

Tam, C. K. W. (1969). The drag on a cloud of spherical particles in low Reynolds number flow. *J. Fluid Mech.* **38**, 537.

Wang, H. & Skalak, R. (1969). Viscous flow in a cylindrical tube containing a row of spherical particles. *J. Fluid Mech.* **38,** 75.

Weibel, E. R. (1962). *Histochemie* **57**, 642.

Whitmore, R. L. (1968) *Rheology of the Circulation*, p. 133. Pergamon Press, Oxford.

Wiederhielm, C. A. (1968). Dynamics of transcapillary fluid exchange. *J. Gen. Physiol.* **52**, suppl. pt. 2, 29s.

Yen, R. T. & Fung, Y. C. (1977). Inversion of Fahraeus effect and effect of mainstream flow on capillary hematocrit. *J. Appl. Physiol.* **42 (4)**, 578.

Chapter 6

Azuma, T. & Hasegawa, M. (1971). A rheological approach to the architecture of arterial walls. *Japan. J. Physiol.* **21**, 27.

Azuma, T. & Oka, S. (1971). Mechanical equilibrium of blood vessel walls. *Amer. J. Physiol.* **221**, 1310.

Bergel, D. H. (1961). The static elastic properties of the arterial wall. *J. Physiol.* **156**, 445.

Burton, A. C. (1951). On the physical equilibrium of the small blood vessels. *Amer. J. Physiol.* **164**, 319.

Burton, A. C. (1972). *Physiology and Biophysics of the Circulation*, 2nd edn., p. 64. Year Book Medical Publishers, Chicago.

Chu, B. M. & Oka, S. (1973). Influence of longitudinal tethering on the tension in thick-walled blood vessels in equilibrium. *Biorheology* **10**, 517.

Cox, R. H. (1979). Regional, species, and age related variations in the mechanical properties of arteries. *Biorheology* **16**, 85.

Fung, Y. C. (1968). Biomechanics. Its scope, history, and some problems of continuum mechanics in physiology. *Appl. Mech. Revs.* **21**, 1.

Fung, Y. C., Fronek, K. & Patitucci, p. (1979). Pseudoelasticity of arteries and the choice of its mathematical expression. *Amer. J. Physiol.* **237 (5)**, H620.

Hayashi, K., Handa, H., Nagasawa, S., Okumura, A. & Moritake, K. (1980a). Stiffness and elastic behavior of human intracranial and extracranial arteries. *J. Biomech.* **13**, 175.

Hayashi, K., Nagasawa, S., Naruo, Y., Okumura, A., Moritake, K. & Handa, H. (1980b). Mechanical properties of human cerebral arteries. *Biorheology* **17**, 211.

Moritake, K., Handa, H., Okumura, A., Hayashi, K. & Niimi, H. (1974). Stiffness of cerebral arteries – its role in the pathogenesis of cerebral aneurysms. *Neurologia Medico-Chir.* **14**, part 1, 47.

Niimi, H., Hayashi, K., Sato, M., Handa, H., Moritake, K. & Okumura, A. (1975). Nonlinear theory of pulse waves in blood vessels. *J. Phys. Soc. Japan* **38**, 1516.

Oka, S. (1968). Theoretical studies on hemorheology. The 16th Rheology Symposium, Sapporo, 1967. *Zairyo* **17**, 300 (in Japanese).

Oka, S. (1972). Some theoretical studies on hemorheology. In *Advances in Biophysics*, ed. M. Kotani, vol. 3, p. 97, University of Tokyo Press, Tokyo.

Oka, S. & Azuma, T. (1970). Physical theory of tension in thickwalled blood vessels in equilibrium. *Biorheology* **7**, 109.

Okumura, A., Hayashi, K., Moritake, K., Handa, H., Matsuda, L., Niimi, H. & Toda, N. (1976). Role of vascular smooth muscle in the mechanical properties of arteries. *Proceedings of the 10th International Congress on Angiology*, Tokyo, p. 590.

Patel, D. J., Janicki, J. S. & Carew, T. E. (1969). Static anisotropic elastic properties on the aorta in living dogs. *Circ. Res.* **25**, 765.

Patel, D. J. & Vaishnav, R. N. (1972). The rheology of large blood vessels. In *Cardiovascular Fluid Dynamics*, ed. D. H. Bergel, vol. 2, p. 1. Academic Press, London.

Tanaka, T. T. & Fung, Y. C. (1974). Elastic and inelastic properties of the canine aorta and their variation along the aortic tree. *J. Biomech.* **7**, 357.

Vaishnav, R. N., Young, J. T., Janicki, J. S. & Patel, D. J. (1972). Nonlinear anisotropic elastic properties of the canine aorta. *Biophys. J.* **12**, 1008.

Chapter 7

Aroesty, J. & Gross, J. F. (1972). Pulsatile flow in small blood vessels. I. Casson theory. *Biorheology* **9**, 33.

Gaehtgens, P. (1970). Pulsatile pressure and flow in the mesenteric vascular bed of the cat. *Pflügers Arch.* **316**, 140.

Hale, J. F., McDonald, D. A. & Womersley, J. R. (1955). Velocity profiles of oscillating arterial flow, with some calculations of viscous drag and the Reynolds number. *J. Physiol.* **128**, 629.

Horimoto, M., Koyama, T., Mishina, H. & Asakura, T. (1979). Pulsatile blood flow in arteriole of frog web. *Biorheology* **16**, 163.

Intaglietta, M., Richardson, D. R. & Tompkins, W. R. (1971). Blood pressure, flow and elastic properties in microvessels of the cat omentum. *Amer. J. Physiol.* **221**, 922.

Lamb, H. (1898). On the velocity of sound in a tube, as affected by the elasticity of the walls. *Manchester Mem.* **42**, 1.

McDonald, D. A. (1974). *Blood Flow in Arteries*, 2nd edn. p. 356. Edward Arnold, London.

Morgan, G. W. & Ferranti, W. R. (1955). Wave propagation in elastic tubes filled with streaming liquid. *J. Acoust. Soc. Amer.* **27**, 715.

Noordergraaf, A. (1969). Hemodynamics. In *Biological Engineering*, ed. H. P. Swan, p. 391. McGraw-Hill, New York.

Rappaport, M. B., Bloch, E. H. & Irwin, J. W. (1959). A manometer for measuring dynamic pressure in the microvascular system. *J. Appl. Physiol.* **14**, 651.

Resal, M. H. (1876). Note sur les petits mouvements d'un fluide incompressible dans un tuyau elastique. *J. Math. Pures Appl. Liouville* **2**, 342.

Scott Blair, G. W. (1959). An equation for the flow of blood, plasma and serum through glass capillaries. *Nature* **183**, 613.

Thurston, G. B. (1973). Frequency and shear rate dependence of viscoelasticity of human blood. *Biorheology* **10**, 375.

Thurston, G. B. (1976). The effects of frequency of oscillatory flow on the impedance of rigid, blood-filled tubes. *Biorheology* **13**, 191.

Uchida, S. (1956). The pulsating viscous flow superposed on a steady laminar motion of incompressible fluid in a circular pipe. *ZAMP* **7**, 403.

Weber, W. (1866). Theorie der durch Wasser oder andere inkompressible Flüssigkeiten in elastischen Röhren fortpflanzten Wellen. *Ber. Verhandl. Königl. Sächs. Ges. Wiss.* **18**, 353.

Witzig, K. (1914). Ueber erzwungene Wellenbewegungen zäher, inkompressibler Flüssigkeiten in elastischen Röhren. Ph.D. thesis, University of Bern.

Womersley, J. R. (1955). Oscillatory motion of a viscous liquid in a thin-walled elastic tube. I. The linear approximation for long waves. *Phil. Mag.* **46**, 199.

Womersley, J. R. (1957). Oscillatory flow in arteries: the constrained elastic tube as a model of arterial flow and pulse transmission. *Phys. Med. Biol.* **2**, 178.

Young, T. (1808). Hydraulic investigations. *Phil. Trans.* **98**, 164.

Chapter 8

Adams, C. W. M. & Bayliss, O. B. (1969). The relationship between diffuse intimal thickening, medial enzyme failure and intimal lipid deposition in various human arteries. *J. Atheroscler. Res.* **10**, 327.

Azuma, T. & Fukushima, T. (1976). Flow patterns in stenotic blood vessel models. *Biorheology* **13**, 337.

Carew, T. C. (1973). Ph.D. thesis. In *Atherogenesis: Initiating Factors*, p. 102. Excerpta Medica, Amsterdam.

Caro, C. G., Pedley, T. J., Schroter, R. C. & Seed, W. A. (1978). *The Mechanics of the Circulation*, Oxford University Press.

Caro, C. G. (1978). Mechanics and mass transport of the arterial wall. *INSERM* **78**, 33.

Chien, S. (1976). Significance of macrorheology and microrheology in atherogenesis. *Ann. N.Y. Acad. Sci.* **275**, 10.

Copley, A. L. (1974). Hemorheological aspects of the endothelium–plasma interface, *Microvasc. Res.* **8**, 192.

Copley, A. L. (1979). Fibrin (ogen), platelets and a new theory of atherogenesis. *Thrombosis Res.* **14**, 249.

Dintenfass, L. (1964). Viscosity and clotting of blood in venous thrombosis and coronary occlusions. *Circ. Res.* **14**, 1.

Forrester, J. H. & Young, D. F. (1970a). Flow through a converging-diverging tube and its implications in occlusive vascular disease–I. Theoretical development. *J. Biomech.* **3**, 297.

Forrester, J. H. & Young, D. F. (1970b). Flow through a converging–diverging tube and its implications in occlusive vascular disease. II. Theoretical and experimental results and their implications. *J. Biomech.* **3**, 307.

Fox, J. A. & Hugh, A. E. (1966). Localization of atheroma: theory based on boundary layer separation. *British Heart J.* **28**, 388

Fry. D. L. (1973). Responses of the arterial wall to certain physical factors. In *Atherogenesis: Initiating Factors*, p. 93. Excerpta Medica, Amsterdam.

Gessner, F. B. (1973). Hemodynamic theories of atherogenesis. *Circ. Res.* **33**, 259.

Hiramoto, Y. (1969). Mechanical properties of the protoplasm of the sea urchin egg. II. Fertilized egg. *Exp. Cell Res.* **56**, 209.

Hiramoto, Y. (1970). Rheological properties of sea urchin eggs. *Biorheology* **6**, 201.

Johshita, T., Sakata, N., Yoshida, K., Yoshida, Y. & Ooneda, G. (1978).

Arterial circumferential tension and atherosclerosis–adaptation of arterial wall to elevated intravascular pressure and its failure. *J. Jap. Coll. Angiol.* **18**, 912 (in Japanese).

Kamiya, N. & Kuroda, K. (1958). Studies on the velocity distribution of the protoplasmic streaming in the myxomycete plasmodium. *Protoplasma* **49**, 1.

Kandarpa, K. & Davids, N. (1976). Analysis of the fluid dynamic effects on atherogenesis at branching sites, *J. Biomech.* **9**, 735.

Karino, T., Kwong, H. H. M. & Goldsmith, H. L. (1979). Particle flow behaviour in models of branching vessels. I. Vortices in 90° T-junctions. *Biorheology* **16**, 231.

Karnowsky, J. J. (1967). Ultrastructural basis of capillary permeability studied with peroxidase as a tracer. *J. Cell Biol.* **35**, 213.

Lee, J. S. & Fung, Y. C. (1971). Flow in nonuniform small blood vessels. *Microvasc. Res.* **3**, 272.

Matsuda, I., Niimi, H., Moritake, K., Okumura, A. & Handa, H. (1978). The role of hemodynamic factors in arterial wall thickening in the rat. *Atherosclerosis* **29**, 363.

Matunobu, Y. & Arakawa, M. (1974). Model experiment on the post-stenotic dilation in blood vessels. *Biorheology* **11**, 457.

Merrill, E. W., Cokelet, G. C., Britten, A. & Wells, R. E. Jr. (1963). Non-Newtonian rheology of human blood – effect of fibrinogen reduced by 'subtraction'. *Circ. Res.* **13**, 48.

Merrill, E. W., Gilliland, E. R., Lee, T. S. & Salzman, E. W. (1966). Blood rheology: effect of fibrinogen deduced by addition. *Circ. Res.* **18**, 437.

Miller, I. R., Graet, H. & Frei, Y. F. (1973). Cholesterol exchange between surface layers and plasma proteins in bulk. In *Atherogenesis: Initiating Factors*, p. 251. Excerpta Medica, Amsterdam.

Mitchell, J. R. A. & Schwartz, C. J. (1965). *Arterial Disease*. Blackwell Scientific Publishers, Oxford.

Nakache, M. & Péronneau, P. (1979). Relationship between hydrodynamic forces and vascular wall phenomena – II. Study of the influence of friction on the parietal microenvironment by the fixed enzyme method. *Biorheology* **16**, 265.

Nerem, R. M., Mosberg, A. T. & Schwerin, W. D. (1976). Transendothelial transport of ^{131}I-albumin. *Biorheology* **13**, 71.

Niimi, H. (1979). Role of stress concentration in arterial walls in atherogenesis. *Biorheology* **16**, 223.

Niimi, H., Horie, R., Yamori, Y. & Oka, S. (1979). Hemodynamic factors on the development of atherogenesis in stroke-prone SHR. *Jap. Heart J.* **20**, (suppl. 1), 368.

Niimi, H., Kawano, Y., Hayashi, K., Handa, H., Moritake, K. Okumura, A. & Matsuda, I. (1976). Hemodynamic study on pathogenesis of atherosclerosis – flow characteristics in arterial bifurcation. *Proceedings of the 10th International Congress on Angiology* Tokyo, p. 595.

Niimi, H. & Oka, S. (1979). Regional stress and deformation in an aneurysmal dilation of arterioles. *Microvasc. Res.* **17**, no. 3, S4.

Niimi, H. & Yamakawa, T. (1980). Fine structure of blood flow near an atherosclerotic plaque-like wall. *2nd International Congress on Mechanics in Medicine and Biology*, p. 130.

Oka, S. (1976). A theoretical approach to the effect of shear stress on the development of atheroma. *Thrombosis Res.* **8** (suppl. 2), 305.

Oka, S. (1979). Physical theory of permeability of vascular walls in relation to atherogenesis. *Biorheology* **16**, 203.

Palade, G. E. & Bruns, R. R. (1968). Structural modulations of plasmalemmal vesicles, *J. Cell Biol.* **37**, 633.

Renkin, E. M. (1964). Transport of large molecules across capillary walls. *Physiologist* **7**, 20.

Rodbard, D. & Chrambach, A. (1970). Unified theory for gel electrophoresis and gel filtration. *Proc. Nat. Acad. Sci.* **65**, 970.

Ross, R. & Glomset, J. A. (1976). The pathogenesis of atherosclerosis, *New England J. Med.* 295, 369, 420.

Schmid-Schönbein, G. W., Fung, Y. C. & Zweifach, B. W. (1975). Vascular endothelium–leukocyte interaction. *Circ. Res.* **36**, 173

Seifriz, W. (1924). The structure of protoplasm and of inorganic gels. *Br. J. Exp. Biol.* **1**, 431.

Simionescu, M., Simionescu, N. & Palade, G. E. (1975). Segmental differentiations of cell junctions in the vascular endothelium. The microvasculature. *J. Cell Biol.* **67**, 863.

Smith, R.L. Blick E.F., Coalson, J. & Stein, P.D. (1972). Thrombus production by turbulence. *J. Appl. Physiol.* **32**, 261.

Stein, P. D. & Sabbah, H. N. (1974). Measured turbulence and its effect on thrombus formation. *Circ. Res.* **35**, 608.

Stein, P. D., Sabbah, H. N., Anbe, D. H. & Walburn, F. J. (1979). Blood velocity in the abdominal aorta and common iliac artery of man. *Biorheology* **16**, 249.

Texon, M., Imparato, A. M., Helpern, M. (1965). Role of vascular dynamics in the development of atherosclerosis. *JAMA* **194**, 168.

Weinbaum, S. (1979). Theoretical models of vesicular transport and endothelial membrane interaction. *Biorheology* **16**, 297.

Wesolowski, S. A., Fries, E. C., Sabin, A. M. & Sawyer, P. N. (1965). Significance of turbulence in hemic systems and in the distribution of the atherosclerotic lesion. *Surgery* **57**, 155.

Wissig, S. L. (1979). The role of endothelial clefts in the permeability of capillaries and venules to protein. Abstract, *2nd World Congress on Microcirculation*, p. 21.

Young, D. F. & Tsai, F. Y. (1973). Flow characteristics in models of arterial stenoses – I. Steady flow. *J. Biomech.* **6**, 395.

Yu, S. K. & Goldsmith, H. L. (1973). Behavior of model particles and blood cells at spherical obstructions in tube flow. *Microvasc. Res.* **6**, 5.

Index

asbolute dynamic modulus, 23
active tension, 114–15
aneurysmal dilation, 186–7
apparent viscosity, 9
atherogenesis, 163
atherosclerosis, 163
ATP content, 82–3
attenuation, 143–6, 149
axial accumulation, 48

Bernoulli's equation, 151
biorheology, 2
Basius' formula, 15
blood, 28–9
   nonlinear viscoelasticity of, 37
   non-Newtonian viscosity of, 33–4
   thixotropy of, 34
   viscoelasticity of, 35–7
   viscosity of, 38–40
blood clots, 60
   viscoelasticity of, 61–3
blood rheology, 28
   at near-zero gravity, 63–4
   and clinical medicine, 65–6
blood vessels, 111
   pseudoelasticity of, 137
   shape of, 139–40
   viscoelasticity of, 135–7
   walls of, 111–14, 140
bolus flow, 102–6
bulk modulus, 20

capillary-tissue fluid exchange, 98–102
cardiac output, 138–9
cardiovascular system, 3
Casson's equation, 40, 42
Casson fluid, 40–6
Casson plot, 40, 41
Casson viscosity, 41
Casson yield stress, 41, 42–4
central packing, 77
centrifugal core, 46
cholesterol content, of red cell
   membrane, 83

circumferential tension, 114
coefficient of resistance, 15
complex modulus, 24
complex velocity, 143
complex viscosity, 24, 148
compressibility of fluid, 7
constitutive equation, 1, 127
constricted tube, flow in, 151–7
Copley–Scott Blair phenomenon, 57–60, 66
cortex, 176
Couette flow, 7, 8
counter-rotating rheoscope, 74–5
creep, 136
critical Reynolds number, 13

Darcy's constant, 99
Darcy's law, 99
   generalized, 101
deformation, 6
diabetes, 109
diastolic pressure, 138
diffusion, activation energy for, 173
diffusion coefficient, 172–3
Dintenfass' equation, 39
dissipation of mechanical energy, 16
dynamic incremental strain, 126–7
dynamic incremental stress, 126–7
dynamic modulus, 22, 23
dynamic viscoelasticity, 22–4
dynamic viscosity, 24

Einstein's equation, 17
ektacytometer, 75–7
elastic modulus, 19–20
elastic tension, 114–15
electric double layer, 66, 189, 192
elliptocytosis, 86
embolism, 160
embolus, 160
endoplasm, 176

Fahraeus effect, 54–5
Fahraeus–Lindqvist effect, 55–7

Index

fiber-arrest method, 78
filtration constant, 88
filtration method, 79–80
floor attachment method, 77
flow rate, 10–12
flow resistance, 53–4
fluid mosaic model, 71
form factor, 18
four-element model, 22

heart rate, 139
hematocrit, 28
  affect on blood viscosity, 38
hemorheology, 2
Hookean solid, 19–20
Hooke's law, 1, 19
hydrostatic pressure, 5
hypertension, 184–5
hypoglycemia, 109–10
hysteresis, 20
  loop, 20

incremental Posisson's ratio, 128
incremental strain, 126
incremental stress, 126
incremental theory, 125
incremental Young's modulus, 127
intermembrane potential, 189

junction, 173, 177
junctional complex, 173

Kelvin model, 21
Krogh's model, 98

laminar flow, 10
Laplace's law, 117–19
loss modulus, 22, 23

macroglobulinemia, 66
macromolecular pathways, 171–5
magnetic particle method, 176
mass transfer boundary layer, 166
Maxwell model, 21
membrane elasticity, 81, 82
membrane viscoelasticity, 82
microcirculation, 87
  and clinical medicine, 108–10
microhemorheology, 191
micropipette method, 78–9
microrheology, 191
microvessels, 4
Moens–Korteweg formula, 144
molar flux, 171
multiple myeloma, 66

Neo-Hookean elasticity, 131–3
Newtonian flow, 9
Newtonian fluid, 9
Newtonian viscosity, 9
Newton's law of viscosity, 1, 8
non-Newtonian flow, 9
non-Newtonian fluid, 9
normal stress, 5–6

occlusive arterial disease, 84–5
Oka–Azuma equation, 116, 117–20
Oldroyd's effective slip coefficient, 58
oscillatory flow, 141–3
oxygen tension, 83

peaking, 147
pentoxifyllin, 85
permeability, 171–2
permeability area product, 172
phase velocity, 144–5
pinocytosis, 173
plasma, 28
plasma layer, 46
plasma proteins, 38–9
platelet, 28
Poiseuille's law, 12
Poiseuille flow, 12
Poisson's ratio, 20
polycythemia, 65
  smoking as a cause of, 65
post-stenotic dilatation, 157–8
pressure ratio, 117
principal extension ratio, 25
protoplasm, 176
  non-Newtonian viscosity of, 176
  thixotropy of, 176
  viscoelasticity of, 176
pulsatile flow, 138–50, 155–7
  in microvessels, 149–50
pulse, 138
pulse pressure, 138
pulse waves, 139–41, 143–7

radial migration, 48–5
reattachment point, 152
red cells, 28–9
  aggregation of, 29–31
  deformation of, 39–40
  internal viscosity of, 39, 82
  measuring techniques of deformability of, 73–81
  membrane structure of, 71–3
  sedimentation of, 31–3
red cell deformability, 4, 67–8
  and clinical medicine, 85–6

Index

red cell shape, 68–71
relaxation time, 21
retardation time, 21
rheology, 1
rouleaux, 29
Reynolds number, 13

screening effect, 55
sedimentation, 31–3
sedimentation rate, 31
Segré–Silberberg effect, 49
separation, 152
separation point, 152
separation region, 151
serum, 29
7-constant theory, 131
shear, 8
shear modulus, 20
shear rate, 8
shear stress, 8
shear-thickening, 9
shear-thinning, 9
sheet flow, 106–8
sickle cell disease, 86
sigma effect, 56
sludging, 29
Sobin–Fung model, 107
spectrin, 71
sphericity index, 70, 71
spherocytosis, 86
spin label technique, 80–1
spot welded junction, 173
Starling's hypothesis, 88
steepening, 147
stenosis, 152, 154
stiffness, 134
Stokes' law, 31
Stokes' relation, 11
strain, 5
strain energy, 19
strain energy density function, 24–6, 130
strain invariant, 25
streamline separation, 152
stress, 5
stress concentration, 185–6
stress invariant, 5
stress relaxation, 136
stroke volume, 139

suspension, viscosity of, 15–18
systolic pressure, 138

tangential stress, 5–6
tank tread motion, 68
Taylor factor, 18
telescopic flow, 10
tethering effect, 131, 141, 145
thixotropy, 26–7
 of blood, 34
 of protoplasm, 176
thrombelastograph, 60–1
thrombosis, 160–3
thrombus, 160, 189
tight junction, 173
Toms' phenomenon, 60
tubular pinch effect, 49
turbulence, 157, 162, 164
turbulent flow, 13
 of blood, 85

velocity distribution, 10, 11–14
velocity gradient, 8
velocity profile, 10
vesicle, 174–5
vesicle diffusion theory, 182–4
viscoelasticity, 20–2
 of blood, 35–7
 of blood clots, 61–3
 of blood vessels, 135–7
 of protoplasm, 176
viscometry, 73–4
viscosity, 7
 of blood, 33–4, 38–40
 of blood clots, 60–3
 Newton's law of, 1, 9 ·
 of protoplasm, 176
Voigt model, 21
volume fraction, 17

wall surface effect, 57–60
wave velocity, 143–46
Weibel model, 107
white cells, 28
wholebody vibration, 171, 182
Womersley parameter, 143

Young's modulus, 20

zeta potential, 66

RAYMOND H. FOGLER LIBRARY
DATE DUE

SUBJECT TO
WEEKS